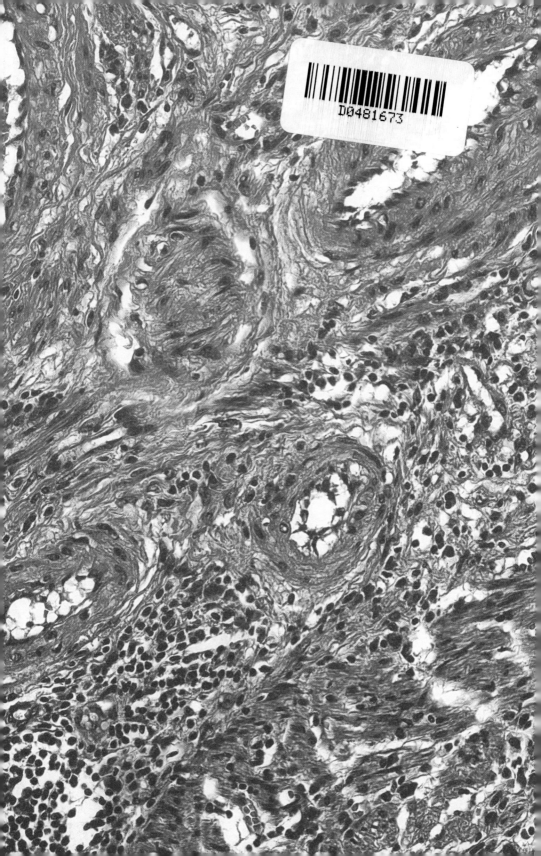

DAUGHTER

of

FAMILY G

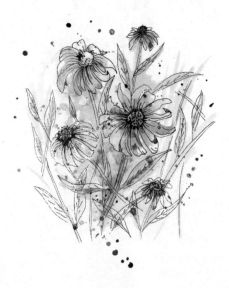

Ami McKay

DAUGHTER

of

FAMILY G

A Memoir of Cancer Genes,
Love and Fate

ALFRED A. KNOPF CANADA

PUBLISHED BY ALFRED A. KNOPF CANADA

Copyright © 2019 Ami McKay

www.penguinrandomhouse.ca

Knopf Canada and colophon are registered trademarks.

Library and Archives Canada Cataloguing in Publication
Title: Daughter of Family G.: a memoir of cancer genes, love and fate / Ami McKay.
Names: McKay, Ami, 1968- author.
Identifiers: Canadiana (print) 20190080795 | Canadiana (ebook) 20190080833 | ISBN 9780345809469 (hardcover) | ISBN 9780345809483 (HTML)
Subjects: LCSH: McKay, Ami, 1968- | LCSH: McKay, Ami, 1968-—Health. | LCSH: McKay, Ami, 1968-—Family. | LCSH: Genetic disorders—Patients—Canada—Biography. | LCSH: Cancer—Patients—Canada—Biography. | LCSH: Authors, Canadian—Biography. | CSH: Authors, Canadian (English)—Biography
Classification: LCC PS8625.K387 A3 2019 | DDC C818/.603—dc23

Text and cover design by Kelly Hill

Photo on page 30 courtesy of Howard Romero;
all other photos courtesy of Ami McKay

Endpapers: ©Ami McKay "Pauline's Gift 1919," a magnified detail of a reconditioned pathology slide from the University of Michigan Department of Pathology Archives.

Interior images: pg 11, *3800 Early Advertising Cuts*, pg 57, *Pictorial Archive of Decorative Frames and Labels*, both from Dover Pictorial Archive Series; all other images courtesy of Shutterstock: (firework emoji) kornn; (all other emojis) Carboxylase; (parchment) design36; (frames) Rangizzz; Alberto Masnovo

Printed and bound in Canada

10 9 8 7 6 5 4 3 2 1

Penguin
Random House
KNOPF CANADA

For Ian and the boys

CONTENTS

III

Hope. Trust. Dream.

I am out
with lanterns,
looking for
myself.

—Emily Dickinson

The events in this book are laid out in alternating chapters of history, memory and being. They take place before I was born; in my past; and during the year I spent writing it. I hope that by weaving the timelines together, rather than placing them end-to-end, I have helped to reveal threads of understanding and truth between the generations.

Although a memoir, by definition, relies heavily on the author's memory, I have made every effort to verify and support the details of this work. Every page is informed by facts gleaned from various sources—medical records, conference reports, scientific journals, personal diaries, photographs, letters, newspaper articles, pathology slides, interviews, census schedules, city directories, genealogical pedigrees, death certificates, obituaries and wedding announcements. Throughout, I kept my eye on bringing clarity, truth and authenticity to the personal stories that are the driving force behind this book.

Whenever it was possible, I interviewed family members, medical practitioners and genetic researchers via email, by phone or in person, including conducting conversations with Dr. Henry T. Lynch, the "father of hereditary cancer detection and prevention," and Dr. Bert Vogelstein, director of the Ludwig Cancer Research Center at Johns Hopkins University.

I have, to the best of my knowledge, been truthful in my portrayal of both the living and the dead. And, without doubt, I have freely shared the innermost workings of my fiercely sincere, though imperfect, heart.

In My Blood

One week after 9/11, I walk into a hospital in rural Indiana and ask a nurse to draw six vials of blood from my arm. I need to know what the future holds, at least my meagre part of it. I'm a healthy, thirty-three-year-old mother of two who can't stop thinking about what tomorrow might bring.

A small TV perched on a filing cabinet in the nurse's office is tuned to the morning news. A commentator with perfect hair and straight teeth stares at me from the screen. The crawl beneath her smiling face reads: IS THIS THE NEW NORMAL?

The nurse, prepping her kit, asks, "Will this make you squeamish?"

"No. I'll just look away."

I don't. I watch every step of the procedure from start to finish—the elastic band pulling tight around my arm, the nurse's fingers prodding for a vein, the slip of the needle into my skin, the steady flow of dark red blood into each tube as the nurse deftly swaps them, one after another—*one, two, three, four, five, six.* I'm looking to see if I can spot the ghosts in my blood.

Within the hour, the samples are shipped to a lab at a university in Nebraska. Researchers there will search for a genetic mutation in my DNA that predisposes me to developing several types of cancer. It's a terrifying list. Colon. Endometrial. Ovarian. Stomach. Bile duct. Liver. Kidney. Pancreas. Upper urinary tract. Brain. Small intestine. Breast. Skin. The literature from the lab says: *A far greater than average risk, at an earlier than average age.* My uncle was diagnosed with his first cancer at twenty-six, my grandmother at fifty, her brother at forty-nine, her sister at forty-three, my mother at fifty-eight. Mom joked and said it was the first time in her life that she'd been a late bloomer. Cancer occurs so frequently in my family, it's become a cruel rite of passage. The list of known initiates dates back to 1856.

The method the lab will use to test my blood is the latest in medical technology, but pathologists and geneticists have been studying my family for well over a century, working to make sense of a disease that's haunted us for generations. We are the longest and most detailed cancer genealogy ever studied in the world. Science needs us as much as we need it.

Several months later, I have a phone conversation with Dr. Henry T. Lynch to get my results. He's the chair of the Department of Preventive Medicine at Creighton University, head of the lab where my blood was tested, and the man for whom the cancer syndrome my family suffers from was named. He's also someone my discerning, no-nonsense mother considers to be an honorary member of our family. In her estimation, "Henry's a saint."

After we exchange greetings, Dr. Lynch says, "I want to thank you and the members of your family for helping us all these years." His voice is cheerful and grandfatherly, which makes for lovely chitchat, but it also makes his explanation about the implications of having Lynch syndrome strangely unnerving. "The lifetime risk for certain cancers increases at an extraordinary rate compared to the general population, so having the mutation puts one in the category of what we call 'accelerated carcinogenesis,' that is, rapid evolution of cancer." He tells me if I have the genetic marker, there's an 85 percent chance I'll get colon cancer in my lifetime and there's nothing I can do to prevent it. No amount of meditation or healthy foods or exercise can stop it.

My stomach tightens. Even though I've known all those things for quite some time, hearing it straight from Henry makes it seem new and alarming. *Rapid evolution of cancer.* And he hasn't even gotten to my results.

We converse at length about my mom and my uncle and my grand-mother, folding their cancer milestones into our small talk. It feels like catching up with an old friend.

I mention other relatives, not by name but by their relationship to me, and their age at the onset of cancer—people who died long before I was born, people whose medical records Henry knows intimately. I need him to know that I, too, have a vast knowledge of their suffer-ing. I've always been an A student. I want him to see how hard I've studied for a test that I can't ace.

When he finally gets around to delivering the news, his voice cracks and falters. "Well, I really feel badly telling you this, but you *did* inherit the gene. You *do* have the mutation."

There's sympathy there, and heartbreak—his and mine.

"And now, by God," he adds, "I want you to have a colonoscopy as soon as possible. I truly hope everything will turn out okay."

"Thanks, Dr. Lynch. I'll get on it right away." Even though I'd told myself a hundred times over it would probably turn out this way, I'm completely devastated. I do my best not to cry as I listen to the rest of what he's got to say.

"Just as the risk of developing colorectal cancer in your lifetime is extremely high, the same goes for endometrial cancer. I urge you to contact a doctor immediately if you experience any unusual pain or symptoms." One by one he lists the annual screenings, tests, scopes and procedures I'll require, along with prophylactic surgeries I should consider having, soon.

From this moment on, I'll never "not know" again. I now live in an unsettling state between wellness and cancer. I am an unaffected carrier, a "previvor."

This is my new normal.

When science offered me the chance to glimpse my future, I took it. What it didn't show me was how to live with what I saw. By the time I received my results, I'd witnessed the wreckage of cancer in my family several times over. I'd lost people I loved, admired and adored. How was I to cope with knowing that same fate lurks in my blood?

As a child, I listened to the women in my family tell stories of the past—grandmothers, aunts and cousins sitting around the kitchen table with my mother, sometimes laughing until they cried, sometimes sobbing through words of grief. They spoke of relatives who lived before I was born—people who came from nothing, who faced great hardship, who died too young. The women in those tales stared down death, looked after the sick, and conversed with fate. They spread the truth through story, even when others didn't wish to hear it.

This is how I learned that stories have power—to make sense of the world, to give voice to dreams, to nurture hope and banish fear.

What I didn't know then was that those stories would provide me with what I need to navigate life with Lynch syndrome. Sometimes the best advice on how to live comes from listening to the dead.

I am now fifty.

My sons are young men.

My mother and the women who sat around her table are gone.

This book is my attempt to keep their stories alive as I come to terms with what lies ahead.

Looking to the same place science has gone for answers—to my ancestors, my family, my blood—I wrote my way between their past and my present, chasing after lost voices in hopes of finding mine.

It was a journey that revealed truths shared across generations, and secrets hidden in stacks of worn journals and yellowed papers. Each discovery led to another, creating a twisted path of revelations that wound between old homesteads and graveyards; research laboratories and hospital archives; groundbreaking scientists and long-lost family. Every encounter brought new connections and stories, and with them came a new narrative of understanding.

The world is now a place where facts and information are at our fingertips. Genomes are regularly sequenced to "find your heritage" or "understand your DNA." Current research shows that one out of every 279 people has Lynch syndrome. Yet only 5 percent have been diagnosed. A simple spit test can determine a myriad of health concerns a person will likely need to address in their lifetime. A new era in medicine has arrived.

Information is power, science says. *It saves lives.*

Yes, absolutely it does.

And our stories keep us whole.

There is probably
no other instance
in which one family
has contributed so
much understanding
of an important
genetic disease
such as this.

—H.T. Lynch, MD, chair of the Department of
Preventive Medicine, Creighton University

Wish. Myth. Curse.

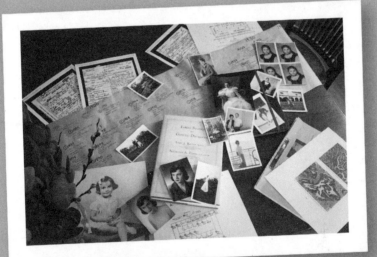

I.

Not Yet

Scots Bay, Nova Scotia, July 2017

I'm standing on the back porch of a seaside farmhouse, surrounded by friends. The evening breeze off the Bay of Fundy is cool and damp, but not unkind. It feels more like September than late July. Melancholy. Bittersweet. It's my birthday—forty-nine.

A few of us lean against the lichen-checked railing while the rest of the guests mingle around a bonfire in the yard. The window above the kitchen sink is open, and I hear water running, someone washing dishes, clanking pots and pans. It's my eldest son. "Don't worry about that right now," I tell him through the screen. "It can wait." He gives me a goofy grin, pretends he can't hear me. Later, the kitchen will be spotless, as if the party never happened. Happy birthday to me.

I stretch my arm out from under the roof of the porch and catch wet in the palm of my hand. It's starting to rain but no one seems to mind. The bonfire hisses and cracks. My two old barn cats are curled on a faded lawn chair, tucked in a knot of mutual comfort. One, pale ginger, the other, tortoiseshell calico. Yin and Yang. Yin stretches, his claws grasping at nothing, then opens his mouth in a wide toothy yawn. Not a care in the world. Someone brings out a guitar and we porch dwellers start to sing Fleetwood Mac's "Landslide," our voices courting coyote song as daylight fades. The lyrics catch me off guard, threaten to make me cry. *Shit.* I think. *Forty-nine.* The child in my heart doesn't know if she can handle it.

My eldest brother was fifty.

My other brother was thirty-nine.

One of my cousins was thirty-seven.

Another, fifty-one.

Our generation hasn't escaped cancer's reach.

My husband takes my hand, gives it a gentle squeeze, leads me into the house. "Time for cake." He is my heart, my haven, my best friend. Later, when the house is silent and dark, he'll still be at my side. I hope he can't see the tears in my eyes.

A crowd of smiling faces gathers around me, laughing, singing, the kitchen awash with flickering candlelight. My big brother, the survivor, sings louder than the rest. *Happy birthday, dear Ami . . .* My son sneaks a fingerful of frosting from the edge of the cake and gives me a sly wink. I scowl in fake disapproval, then do the same, on behalf of his little brother who's away at summer camp. Family traditions mean everything.

Happy birthday to you . . .

Closing my eyes I blow out the candles, make a wish. It's the same wish I've made every birthday for the past sixteen years, two simple words I hold in my heart: *not yet.*

To pretend cancer won't ever come for me is a dangerous game. Yet somehow this annual ritual of asking it to wait seems reasonable and fair. Anticipating cancer is one thing, negotiating life as I wait for its arrival, another. Fear has become both enemy and friend. It can eat me alive. It can save my life.

I pray my bargain with fate will last another year.

2.

Afternoons with Alice

Lebanon, Indiana, 1980

The summer I turn twelve, people start leaving. Both of my brothers and my sister get married and move out. My grandfather suddenly passes away in his sleep. "At least it wasn't cancer," my grandmother says, emphatically and often. "Thank God for that." She speaks from experience and wants everyone to know it. Family. Friends. Strangers. The Avon lady. The mailman. "I had colon cancer, twice, before I hit sixty. Next time the Big C comes around, I'm sure it'll do me in." She's seventy-five.

She lives in a mobile home parked in our backyard, steps away from the only place I've ever called home. It's a fairly recent arrangement, and my mom isn't wild about it. The spot where the trailer sits was formerly a garden, and our solid limestone ranch house, my mom's sanctuary, down a country lane, away from town and gossip, away from her mother. It'd been the perfect place to settle with my dad and raise a family.

Now, my mom looks out the kitchen window before she dares step out the back door, makes mad dashes to fill the bird feeder, doesn't bother to trim her rosebushes for fear she'll get snagged by my grandmother's thorny complaints. Proximity has turned the emotional divide that's long existed between them into the Grand Canyon of Dysfunction.

Frail and hunched, my grandmother is usually cranky, tired and looking for attention. Every case of indigestion or stitch in her side makes her panic. She's constantly thinking she should call the doctor. My mother listens, assesses the situation, then talks her down as best she can. Doctor visits are expensive, especially for things that are only in your head. My grandmother's body may be weak, but her obsession with illness is relentless, Herculean, petulant.

Behind closed doors, my mom begins to refer to my grandmother by her first name. "Alice is at it again," she says to my father while recounting her day. Sometimes my dad makes a joke, tries to get Mom to laugh. Sometimes he knows it's best not to say anything at all. *Alice* becomes a synonym for fretting, whining and occasional deceit. "Don't you dare pull an Alice on me," Mom grumbles, especially when she thinks I'm up to no good. "I won't have it."

I become their go-between. The walk across our backyard is a high-wire act, with my practical, strong-willed mother at one end and fretful Alice at the other. Seeing my grandmother's fragility, my sympathy naturally goes to her. If that bothers my mother, she doesn't say so. She never discourages me from spending time with Alice, never tells me not to love her, never pulls me into their fights. The only warning she gives is this: "Take whatever your grandmother says with a grain of salt."

"Why?"

"She likes to pretty-up the truth."

"You mean she lies."

"Yes."

The lies are worth the risk. In exchange for reading Alice a few chapters of Agatha Christie's *And Then There Were None*, I'm given a front-row seat to whatever's on her mind. Tucked in the corner of a faded loveseat in her tiny front room, I keep my end of the bargain, then wait for the curtain to rise on her cloudy brown eyes. This is when the stories begin. Crossing my fingers, I pray our conversation will turn to tales of her youth, and talk of hooch, booze and bathtub gin.

Cigarette smoke wafts from a cockeyed ashtray atop a brass stand next to Alice's chair, shrouding my grandmother's motley collection of antiques. Every lamp, figurine, bowl, candlestick, vase, pitcher and teacup is chipped, lopsided, glued, cracked and flawed beyond repair. Little of it is related to our family in any meaningful way. My grandfather bought most of it at estate auctions and flea markets, in hopes of giving their lives an air of grand history, rudely interrupted. The truth is, his hunger for excess left them wanting and poor.

"Your grandfather and I had two weddings," Alice boasts, lighting a second Pall Mall Red before her first has expired. "We met in secret and eloped. We were married for over a year before anyone knew what we'd done." Horn-rimmed glasses sliding down her nose, she smirks like a naughty child.

Lifting the lid off a glass candy dish, she offers me a sweet—chocolate mints wrapped in silver foil, butterscotch disks twisted in gold cellophane, sugary jewels of temptation glinting in the late afternoon sun. "Take as many as you like." The overture has begun. I'm no longer her granddaughter, but audience, confidante, conspirator.

"Didn't your parents like Grampy?" I ask, unwrapping a mint and popping it into my mouth. I'm thinking of the boy my sister, Lori, married fresh out of high school in June. He hadn't grown up in our town and my parents barely knew his family. They'd come to accept him, of course, but there were plenty of questions to go around while they made up their minds.

"My folks liked him just fine," Alice says, daintily picking a bit of tobacco from her lip. "It was your grandfather's parents who objected. They didn't think I was cut from the right cloth."

Decades later, while sifting through newspaper archives and genealogical records, I'll discover the depth of their hypocrisy. My grandfather's mother had been removed from her parents' custody after her mother had been accused of poisoning several relatives, including her abusive husband. My grandfather's father, despite his privileged upbringing, had never held down a steady job, preferring instead to drift between elderly relatives in hopes of being included in their wills. Whereas Alice's own paternal lineage is littered with lords and ladies, leading clear back to William the Conqueror, and her maternal line is populated by hardworking German immigrants who were among the first to establish farms in southeast Michigan.

"Did they ever come around?" I ask, certain I haven't heard the whole story.

"Not exactly. My parents arranged a spectacular second wedding for us, called in every favour they were owed around town, and your grandfather's parents still complained at every turn. Nothing was ever good enough for them. We didn't let that spoil our day, though. I wore a beautiful gown of ivory silk taffeta and your grandfather wore tails. My four sisters were dressed in crepe, the shades of Spanish tile. The chapel was decorated front to back with candles, woodbine and autumn flowers—zinnias, dahlias, marigolds and the like." Alice rests her feet on a low footstool as she basks in the memory, her nylon knee-highs wearily slouched around her swollen ankles.

My dog starts barking outside, which means my dad's home from work. As daylight fades, so does the contentment in Alice's face. She takes a drag on her cigarette and asks, "Do you think a person can go to hell for wanting to die?"

The question doesn't surprise me. Talk of tragedy, loss and death comes easy to her. She relishes turning from light to dark on a dime. Imagine Miss Marple without any mysteries to solve.

I shake my head and shrug, hoping that will be enough.

She stares at me.

"Do I really have to answer?"

"Yes."

Barely a month has passed since she'd threatened to take what remained of my grandfather's prescription meds and "end it." My mother had promptly responded by yanking all the bottles of expired medications from Alice's cupboards. I'd been enlisted to hold the garbage bag.

"Is this person planning on doing something about it?" I ask, testing the waters.

"No. Just wishing she could."

"That's some wish."

"Yes," Alice says. "I'm tired." Seeing the worry on my face she adds, "It would be nice to know when I'm gonna go, that's all. I'm sick of wondering."

There's no sense arguing with her. There never is.

Leaning forward in her chair, Alice reaches for my hand and stares into my eyes. "My aunt Pauline foretold her own passing."

"Really?" I say, wondering if we've finally reached a lie. "She saw her death before it happened?"

"Oh, yes. She even told a doctor as much, several years before she died."

"And was she right?"

"Right down to the how, when and why."

The hairs on the back of my neck stand up. I'm baffled, enthralled, hooked. I desperately want this strange tale to be true.

"She was quite young when cancer took her. I was your age when she passed." Alice's eyes fill with tears.

"Wasn't there anything the doctors could do?"

The corners of Alice's mouth quiver. "It was too fast. Before we knew it, she was gone." Turning her head, she stares out the window. "You'd better run along home now. Your mom will want a hand with fixing dinner."

Standing next to my mother at the kitchen counter, I peel potatoes while she chops onions. I can't stop thinking about Alice's aunt. "Have you ever heard of a Pauline in your family?"

"Who?" Mom asks, scraping the onions off her cutting board and into a frying pan on the stove. They sizzle in a pool of melted butter.

"Pauline," I repeat, still peeling. The name is wonderfully old-fashioned, and sophisticated to my ears. Maybe Alice was lying. Maybe Pauline never existed.

"My grandma Tillie's sister was named Pauline. Is that who you mean?"

I picture Pauline with an angel at her bedside whispering in her ear. "Is it true she predicted her own death?"

Mom plops a slippery potato into a pot half-full of water. "That's how the story goes."

"An *Alice* story or a real story?"

"Oh, it's real. Tillie told it to me when I was young, and she was honest as they come."

My mom is too. She doesn't lie, ever. She has a confidence that never wavers and an unshakable dedication to speaking the truth, even when she knows other people don't want to hear it. I want more than anything to be like her.

"How did Pauline see her passing? Did she have some sort of vision? Was she a fortune teller? A witch?"

"Is that what *she* told you?" my mom asks, gesturing towards my grandmother's house with her knife.

"No. She didn't say anything like that." The last thing I want is to start an argument between them.

Setting her knife on the counter, my mother takes a deep breath. "Jesus, poor Pauline. I'd almost forgotten about her."

"But was she?" I press.

"Was she what?"

"A witch?"

"God no. She was a dressmaker."

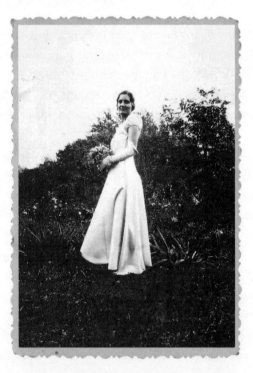

Alice on her "official" wedding day, 1931

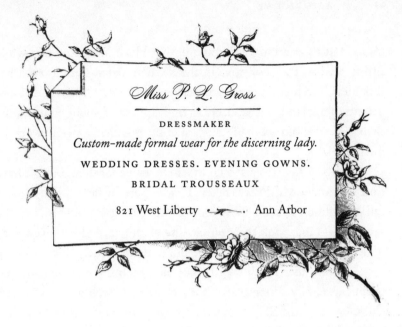

3·

The Dressmaker and Fate

Ann Arbor, Michigan, 1895

Pauline Gross walks along a stone path that winds through Forest Hill Cemetery. She pulls a wool shawl around her shoulders as she goes, to guard against the brisk October wind. Except for a lanky university student making his way home from the library, the young dressmaker is alone. Unless, of course, she counts the spirits attached to the rows of tombstones that stretch out before her, former residents of Ann Arbor—great, small, illustrious, meek—hovering close to the remains that rest, facing east, six feet beneath the ground. She swears she can spot them as they skirt among the marble statuary that dots the graveyard—sombre-faced angels, weeping willows, draped urns, and hands pointed towards heaven. *I'm glad they're here*, she thinks. *I'm in the mood for ghosts.*

Brushing a few stray leaves from the seat of a wooden park bench, she sits and waits for twilight, *when the veil is thin between this life and the next.* It's something her grandmother Haab had often said while sitting next to the cookstove in the kitchen, faded quilt around her shoulders, kerchief on her head, grieving over everything she'd lost— parents, homeland, husband, children. Pauline had spent many nights sitting by the old woman's side, silently practicing needlework or mending socks.

"Your mother was just a child when her Vaddr died. I didn't have time to wonder why he was taken. I had to run the farm. I had a house full of children to feed. Now four of them are gone too, dead of the same illness that took their father. The doctors called it cancer. I say it's a curse. I wish I knew what we did to deserve it."

Grandmother Haab had died of old age, but the curse had lived on in the family. Three of Pauline's cousins, as well as her mother's eldest brother, had all died in the past five years. Her cousin Mary had been only thirty-nine.

Who will be next?

The question sets Pauline's heart racing. The unfairness of it all is almost more than she can bear. One day you feel fine, in perfect health, no sign of trouble in the womb or gut. Then it comes, swift and cruel, like the wizened hag Perchta from her grandmother's Swabian folk tales. "If she sees you've done wrong, she'll slit your belly, steal your innards, stuff you with stones and straw, and sew you shut!"

Pauline has been keeping a record of all her kin who have succumbed to the disease. She desperately wants to find some sense in their suffering, some pattern that might lead to an answer. So far, all the exercise has done is feed her fear. Her mother is forty-nine, the same age her aunt Rosina had been when she'd been struck down.

Will she live to see fifty?

"Don't waste your time pondering death," her mother had said when she'd confessed her worries. "It doesn't do anyone any good."

"It hasn't done us any good to ignore it."

"Take comfort in the fact that *our* house hasn't been touched."

Not yet, Pauline had thought.

Since then, she'd kept her thoughts to herself. Her father and six of her brothers have their hands full with the farm. Her other brother,

Emmanuel, lives in town but is busy with his new position as a sales clerk at Mack and Co. Her older sister, Lydia, is pregnant with her third child in as many years, as she and her husband, Jacob, are struggling to make ends meet. Her younger sister, Tillie, with whom she shares a room at a local boarding house, is nineteen, perpetually sunny, and constantly planning for marriage and motherhood. Pauline refuses to do or say anything that might shatter her dreams.

Closing her eyes, she tries to imagine falling in love, having children, growing old. She can't see any of it. They all require a hopefulness she simply doesn't possess. For someone who comes from such a large family, she feels quite alone. *Perhaps that's why I prefer the company of ghosts.*

Last night she'd dreamt Grandmother Haab's spirit was floating over her bed, staring down at her, refusing to speak. She'd woken, filled with dread. Since then, she hasn't been able to stop wondering if she too, is fated to suffer the curse.

Her grandmother used to talk of the secret rituals the women in her village had practiced in order to see their fate—pulling sticks of wood from a pile, dropping molten lead into water, sneaking out to the barn at midnight on the first night of winter to listen to the animals speak. The simplest of the rites had been Pauline's favourite, a ritual to be observed just after the setting of the sun. "You must look to the heavens and wait for your mind to form a thought. If the next sound you hear is the toll of a bell, then you'll know the thought is true. If you hear a dog bark, it's false."

As the last rays of the sun slip low on the horizon, Pauline stares up at a window of open sky.

A lone crow flaps its way to its roost.

One for sorrow, is the first thought that comes to Pauline's mind.

The bells of the library tower begin to peal—mournful, resolute. She has her answer, her fate, her truth. *I'll die before my time.*

Moments later, a gentleman approaches on the path. "Miss Gross!" he calls.

Pauline turns her head, pretending she doesn't see him. She hopes he'll move on, pass her by, not notice her tears.

"Miss Gross," the man says again, drawing near. "I thought it was you."

She discreetly wipes her eyes before facing him. "Good evening, Dr. Warthin."

The doctor touches his hat, gives a slight bow. "*Grüss Gott,*" he says in an attempt at the traditional greeting most Germans use around town.

Pauline had first met the pathologist through Mr. Gottfried Wild, Ann Arbor's finest tailor. In exchange for the use of Wild's sewing machines, Pauline had agreed to take on odd jobs for him, including mending Dr. Warthin's suits. If anyone else had asked this of her she would've taken it as an insult, but Mr. Wild was a master of his craft. "He's a particular one," Mr. Wild had said of the doctor. "With impeccable taste. Not just any old seamstress will do for him."

"I'm not old, and I'm not a seamstress."

"Precisely."

Mr. Wild was from the old country, a friend of the family.

Dr. Warthin was neither, yet he frequented the Swabian quarter of town, most especially Mr. Wild's shop.

Warthin surveys the young dressmaker. "Your cheeks seem rather flushed, Miss Gross. Are you unwell?"

"It's probably just the change in the weather," she says. She's a terrible liar.

Hat in hand, the doctor gestures for her permission to sit next to her on the bench. "May I?"

Pauline nods. He might as well. He's already caught her crying.

Warthin smiles, smooths a wrinkle from the sleeve of his suit coat as he sits. "If something is troubling you, medically or otherwise, I'd gladly hear it and then forget it, if that's what you wish."

She thinks of the trust Mr. Wild puts in her, and of the social gulf that lies between herself and the doctor. Confessing her thoughts to him seems unwise, but she can't recall ever receiving a kinder invitation. Maybe his appearing at the moment of her revelation is also a sign.

Swallowing hard, Pauline says, "I believe I'm going to die before my time."

Warthin doesn't flinch. Doesn't offer up an argument. "A troubling notion."

"My mother says I shouldn't entertain such thoughts."

"The question isn't whether you should or shouldn't, but *why* you do."

"If I tell you why, you'll either think I have good reason, or that I'm dreadfully morbid."

Warthin shakes his head. "By my own choosing I'm surrounded by corpses all day. You can't get more morbid than that."

Pauline's reservations fall away. "People in my family keep dying from the same disease. Dozens of my kin, struck down in the prime of life."

"Consumption," Warthin offers, sure he's got the answer. He's seen it ravage families many times over. He's beginning to believe some families are more susceptible to the disease than others.

"Cancer," Pauline counters. "Of the stomach, intestines and womb. Generation after generation with no end in sight. My late grandmother believed that it was caused by a curse."

"Is that what you believe?"

"I believe in numbers, patterns and details."

Warthin gives a solemn nod. "As do I."

Pauline feels great relief. For the first time in the longest while, she has someone to confide in besides the ghosts.

4.

What We Carry

Scots Bay, Nova Scotia, August 2017
Alice had her version of Pauline's story.

My mother had hers.

Science has one too, as written by Henry T. Lynch et al. in "Historical Aspects of Lynch Syndrome," 2010:

> In 1895 Aldred Warthin, M.D., began his long tenure at the University of Michigan School of Medicine in Ann Arbor. At that time, his seamstress appeared depressed, and being an extremely inquisitive and caring physician, he asked her why she was depressed. She told him it was because she was convinced that she was going to die of cancer and that it would involve her gastrointestinal tract or her female organs, since "Everyone in the family dies of these cancers." This piqued Warthin's interest and he began compiling her pedigree. He found it to be quite alarming, since the very cancers that the seamstress had discussed with him were present through four generations. Also, just as she had predicted, she died at an early age of metastatic endometrial carcinoma. Warthin referred to the pedigree as Family G.

Similar versions of this story have appeared in medical and scientific journals for decades. A kindly doctor volunteers to listen to the woes of a working-class girl, and his act of kindness leads him to a scientific breakthrough that will inform cancer research into the twenty-first century. Aldred S. Warthin, PhD, father of cancer genetics, case closed. But, as most historical anecdotes do, it suffers from man's tendency to erase details for the sake of brevity and for the larger, more pointed goal of creating a hero.

My Pauline, the one I've fashioned here from medical records, historical documents and stories begged from Alice and my mother, is not a nameless seamstress who confessed her woes to a doctor and then vanished into thin air. She was an outspoken and courageous woman who came from a family who loved her. She was intuitive, yes, but also an astute observer of human nature and a stickler for detail. In many ways, for what was to unfold, Warthin needed Pauline far more than she needed him.

From the moment Alice first mentioned Pauline to me, I became obsessed with family history and genealogy, which eventually led me to a career devoted to bringing the stories of forgotten women to light. I lean on Pauline, or at least the idea of her, whenever I'm in need of strength I don't think I possess. I marvel at the fact that she knew her fate and yet didn't let that knowledge destroy her.

That's something I'm still trying to learn.

Out of the blue I get an email from my cousin's daughter, Lacie, who is hoping I can give her information about our family's connection to Lynch syndrome. She's aware of my love of genealogy and that I carry a Lynch syndrome gene. She figures since I keep track of the family tree, I might also keep tabs on our family's medical history. She needs to provide her doctor with a detailed history of cancer in her relatives, so she can undergo genetic testing herself.

> L: I don't know any of this information off the top of my head. The hospital called today asking specifically who had been diagnosed with cancers related to the gene and at what age— grandparents, parents, aunts, uncles, siblings, first cousins. I have no idea about any of it. I told them I would get the info ASAP.

Her grandfather, my uncle Jamie, my mother's brother, had recently died from a Lynch-related cancer. His first cancer diagnosis occurred in his twenties, and his last, number fifteen, when he was seventy-eight. He struggled through surgeries and treatments for fifty years. Colon, stomach, bladder, ureter, rectum . . . the list goes on.

> L: I only met him once. My dad seemed to have a distant relationship with him, and everything about his most recent struggle with cancer I learned from posts I saw on Facebook. I talked to my dad briefly, but he just said 'everyone copes with these things differently,' so I left it at that. Thanks for your help with whatever you can share.

Lacie is in her mid-thirties and mother to a young son. She's scared of what might lie ahead. I know the feeling well. Any parent who carries the mutation has a fifty-fifty chance of passing it on to their children. Her grandfather was, of course, positive for the gene, but Lacie's father has chosen not to get tested. This pisses me off for Lacie and for her child, but I also know how hard it is to make that decision. I shrug off my feelings and focus on what Lacie needs.

> A: I'll pull what I have together for you and send it along. I'm sure this is all a bit unsettling. Sending you love and strength as you go through this process.

Through no fault of hers, Lacie's ties to the family are complicated. As a child, she had little contact with my cousin, her father. She and I stumbled into a friendship only when she spent a summer working in an organic farm co-op in Nova Scotia. Before that, I'd met her just once, in the corridors of a hospital. I was twelve. She was a newborn.

She looks more like me than any of my siblings or cousins. Even my close friends thought she was my sister when they met her. She loves literature and now works in a bookstore. She likes travelling and taking long hikes in the woods. We're more alike than different.

A: One other thing . . . I feel like I should let you know that just because we look alike doesn't mean you have the mutation. It's easy for our hearts and brains to make that leap while going through the testing process. But the researchers always assured me that it doesn't work that way.

I send her a list of names and dates, cancer diagnoses and ages of onset. I include a photo of a hand-drawn family tree that illustrates everyone's relationships to her. I want to be supportive without over-whelming her. I can't imagine what it's like to wonder if you've inher-ited a defective gene from a family you barely know.

A: Call me if you need to talk.

Corresponding with Lacie makes me realize that I need to call my eldest son to find a time when *we* can talk, face to face. He's been living in Halifax since he graduated from art school, an hour and a half away from home. He's busy but happy, actively chasing his dream of being a visual artist, splitting his time between various residencies and art shows. He's just turned twenty-four. He's not yet been tested. He's in love.

He was only eight when I got my test results, so Lynch syndrome and everything that comes with it has been present for most of his life. I've never hidden any of it from either of my sons, believing that being honest and open with them about hereditary cancer is the best way to foster awareness and positive action. I've had conversations with him about the test in the past, and he's said he'll get it done, but after talking with Lacie, I feel as if the clock's sped up—that he needs to do it sooner rather than later. His younger brother is only sixteen and can't get tested for another two years, but he's got no excuse. Until now I'd held back on nudging him to take next steps, but if I don't take it seriously, why should he?

My husband, Ian, volunteers to be the heavy. "I'll lay some fatherly guilt on him, tell him he's making his mother sick with worry."

"Don't joke about it," I say. The mention of illness and the test in the same breath makes me nervous. "You were teasing, right?"

"Sort of," Ian says, wrapping his arms around me. "All I'm saying is I'm willing to be the one to talk to him, if you want."

I can't accept his offer. "No. It needs to come from me."

Our marriage is built on a firm foundation of love, kindness and cooperation. Ian is the problem-solver. I'm the dreamer, always searching for the bigger picture. I know he thinks this task would be easier for him than for me and he wants to take this load off my shoulders. I can't let him.

The next time I'm alone, I pick up my phone to make the call, but instead of dialling my son's number, I cry.

What if I've passed the gene on to my boys?

There's nothing that can change it if I have.

Tears streaming down my face, I think of my mother and wish that I could call her for advice. She always knew the right thing to say. Throughout my adolescence, whenever I'd complained about a tough challenge I'd had to face, she'd put her hand on her hip and proclaim, "Welcome to your next opportunity." That no-nonsense invitation always prompted me to look beyond what I'd seen as a dead end.

Wiping my eyes, I work to turn my blues around. I can't change what fate has handed me or what's inside my sons' DNA. What I can do is honour the best parts of my mom that live inside me, and call my son.

5.

Being Invisible

Lebanon, Indiana, 1974

It's summer. I'm five, almost six, hiding under the kitchen table one night, knobby knees hugged to my chest. A lone firefly clings to the side of the canning jar at my feet. *Blink . . . blink . . . blink.*

The fruity tang of citrus wafts through the air as wedges of lime are sliced on a wooden cutting board and passed around above me. I hear the clink of glasses, the glug and bubble of rum and Coke. The flick of cigarette lighters and the whispery hiss of smoke blown through pursed lips. My mom slips off her white Keds, the rubber edges of their soles squawking. My aunt's sun-kissed shins smell of Coppertone and Enjoli. I connect the dots of the age spots speckled across my grandmother's legs. Starfish. Butterfly. Rabbit. Giraffe.

As I eavesdrop on the enticing world that exists inches above my head, I don't need to see anyone's face. The tone of their voices, the pitch of their laughter, the restless shifting in their seats tells me everything I need to know about their world. Cicada song ratchets through open windows.

I learn that the secret to my grandmother's Jell-O salad is using apple juice instead of water. I learn that my aunt can avoid answering most any question simply by changing the subject. I learn that my mother listens a lot more than she talks.

Before long, their conversation turns to "troubles"—money woes, love gone wrong, someone named Dot who's in grave danger of damaging her reputation.

After Dot's fate is sorted, my grandmother's foot starts tapping. "I have some bad news," she says, her voice hushed. "Jamie's sick again." My uncle, my grandmother's only son.

"Has he gone to the doctor?" my mom asks.

"Had his blood drawn last week, X-rays too. He's waiting on the results."

"Hope it's better news than last time."

The last time it was cancer.

My aunt tries to lighten the mood. "Don't you think Jamie's youngest boy looks just like him?"

"I think he looks more like Uncle Bud," my mom replies. "The spitting image."

My grandmother rotates her ankle until it cracks, then lets out a sigh. Her brother Bud died of multiple cancers at forty-nine, less than two years after winning big in the Irish Sweepstakes.

"All three of them have the same laugh," my aunt says. "Or had, in Bud's case."

I can hear my grandmother sniffing away tears, and then the steady fizz of another round being poured. They clink.

"To Bud."

"To Bud."

"To Bud."

Whose laugh do I have? I wonder. *Who do I take after?*

My grandmother is dramatic, emotional, prone to worry. My aunt is loud and impulsive, the life of the party. My mother is strong, invincible . . . like the lyrics of the Helen Reddy song. *I am woman, hear me roar . . .*

I want to be like her.

I have her dark hair, her slight build, her delicate hands with slender fingers. More than her looks, I want to possess her eye for magic. She masterfully spots stray feathers, shooting stars and four-leaf clovers, all bringers of good luck. She's practical enough to see the world through clear eyes, and courageous enough to believe in miracles.

Don't worry, I tell myself. *Mom is strong. Mom doesn't complain of aches or pains. When she goes to the hospital it's to see other people. Mom doesn't get sick.*

"What if it's worse this time?" my grandmother asks. "What if Jamie doesn't make it?"

"Don't talk that way," my mother says, her tone verging on impatient. "Whatever happens, we'll handle it. Don't assume the worst. Don't tempt fate."

My grandmother wrings her hands in her lap. I can reach out and touch her yellowed fingers if I want to, but I don't.

The ceiling fan begins to *tsk, tsk, tsk, tsk,* scolding her fear.

The firefly flits against the jar's lid trying to escape, *blink . . . blink . . . blink.*

"It's getting late," my aunt says. "Maybe we should call it a night."

After my aunt and grandmother leave, Mom clears the table and washes the dishes. When she's done she pokes her head under the tablecloth and gently flicks me with a dishtowel. "All right, little busybody. Time for bed."

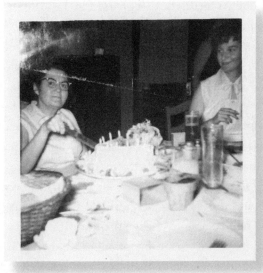

Alice and Mom at the kitchen table on Alice's birthday

6.

Family G

Pauline arrives at three o'clock, as Dr. Warthin had requested, but when she knocks on his office door there's no answer.

Several men in white aprons pass her, giving her sideways looks.

Warthin had said she should wait inside if he happened to be late. "I've an anatomy demonstration beforehand. Sometimes the students' questions go long."

Still, it doesn't feel right to let herself in. If he doesn't arrive soon, she'll leave him a note and go. She checks her watch. *I'll stay until quarter past, no later.*

A couple of orderlies push a gurney up the hallway with a cadaver as cargo, the wheels on the cart chirping in complaint. The cadaver's head lolls towards Pauline, eyes wide, mouth gaping—the first female she's seen since entering the building. Hand to her mouth, she turns away. The orderlies laugh at her, but it isn't the sight of the woman's pale, waxy flesh that unnerves her. It's the men's lack of care of the dead.

Maybe I shouldn't have come here, she thinks. Just because Warthin had shown an interest in what she'd had to say about her family, it didn't mean he'd be able to change their fate.

He certainly hadn't made any promises. All he'd said was that he'd do his best to make sense of their predicament. What more did she expect? At least his interest in her troubles had seemed sincere—a far cry from the doctors who'd thrown up their hands and sent her kin home to die. They'd believed there was no sense in even trying to treat them.

By comparison, Warthin's attention feels miraculous. So much so, that she'd wound up confessing her plan to meet with the doctor to her sister Tillie.

"Is he married?" Tillie had asked.

"No."

"Is he handsome?"

Pauline refused to answer.

"I'll take that as a yes."

So what if he's handsome, Pauline had thought. "I prefer a virtuous man."

"You sound like Mama."

"Good."

Fetching a hatbox from under her bed, Tillie had presented it to Pauline. "You should wear my bonnet with the silk roses on the brim."

"We're not going dancing." Pauline handed the box back. "We're meeting at the university."

Tillie took the bonnet from the box, placed it on her own head, tied the bow under her chin and inspected herself in the mirror. "Who do you think will get married first, you or me?"

"You're the one who snuck a lock of hair into the hem of Lydia's wedding gown," Pauline teased.

In response, Tillie recited a saying their mother had taught them when they were young. "She who wishes to be bride next, must sew her hair into the dress. . . . Don't tell me you've never done it."

"Never."

"Not once?"

Pauline kissed her finger, crossed her heart.

"I'm sorry to have kept you waiting, Miss Gross," Dr. Warthin says, as he rushes towards her and opens the door. "Won't you come in?"

"Thank you," she says, and follows him.

His office is modest. It smells medicinal, faintly perfumed with formaldehyde and ether. A large desk flanked by two chairs takes up most of the space. The desk is covered with an ink-stained blotter and a constellation of scientific paraphernalia—metal forceps, Pasteur pipettes, glass slides, a brass microscope, and a table-top cabinet fitted with shallow drawers meant for holding pathological specimens.

Clearing a stack of books from the chair closest to Pauline, Warthin deposits them on one of the shelves that line the wall behind his desk. "Do have a seat."

As Pauline settles in her chair, she notices that Warthin looks tired. If her mother were there she'd surely say, "He needs sauerkraut, beets, potatoes and liver, to make the blood strong."

Opening her satchel, she produces a few pages of foolscap on which she'd neatly copied the names of family members who'd died from cancer. As the doctor had asked, she'd also included their birth and death dates as well as their relationship to her and other living members of the family, along with any details of their illnesses she could recall. "There are a few details missing," she says, "but I can confirm them with my mother next time I'm home."

Warthin takes the pages from her, then sits behind his desk. "Your family doesn't live in Ann Arbor?"

"Just my brother Emmanuel, my sister Matilda and me. The rest of my family and most of my relatives live in Freedom Township, on land my grandfather settled."

Opening a notebook on his desk Warthin makes notes as he sifts through Pauline's papers. He doesn't speak.

As she waits, Pauline turns her attention to a collection of framed documents hanging next to her on the wall—diplomas peppered with Latin, adorned with ornate calligraphy and gold seals. Perfectly straight, equally spaced, they remind her of the portraits and photographs displayed in the homes of her clients. But there are no touches of home here. No evidence of family. No sweetheart with her eyes on a future with her beloved. The only work of art in the room is a small engraving on yellowed paper, hanging directly below the doctor's lofty credentials. A brass plate affixed to the bottom of its frame reads: *Ritter, Tod und Teufel.* Knight, Death and the Devil.

The knight, in full armour, sits proud on a magnificent steed as he rides through a valley of shadow and decay. He pays no attention to the craggy rocks, dark roots and barren trees. His gaze is set on the path ahead, his goal out of frame. He seems determined, stoic and, Pauline thinks, wholly unaware of the sweet-faced hound racing beside him, desperate to keep pace.

By contrast, Death and the Devil are half-hidden along the roadside, a pair of thorny creatures grown out of the briars and bracken, seeking attention more than prey. Neither looks terribly frightful. To Pauline, they seem barely villains. The Devil is a predictable, goatheaded buffoon. Death, a patient sentinel holding his hourglass aloft, warning passersby of the inevitable.

Unlike the documents around it, the engraving hangs crooked. It's close enough to Pauline that she could reach it. She fights the urge to straighten it.

Looking up from his desk, Warthin notices Pauline's gaze. "I bought it two summers ago at a little shop in Nuremberg on my way to Vienna. Have you ever been?"

"To Nuremberg or Vienna?"

"Either."

"No."

"I keep it here to remind me that it's not enough to understand death, I must also strive to conquer it."

Turning his notebook towards Pauline, he shows her the series of circles and squares he's drawn, connected by several lines. "These represent the members of your family, from your grandfather down to you." He's placed large Xs over the deceased. "Charting the disease in this way is the first step in confirming my suspicions."

"Which are?"

"That your family has an inherited susceptibility to cancer."

She'd already guessed this, but the words still shock her. "What comes after that?" *Please God, let there be something.*

"I'll need to gather more information: death certificates, medical records . . . everything I can concerning the deceased. I'd also like to study the members of your family who are still living. Charting your lives over time may well yield answers as to why the disease is so prevalent. Interviewing as many of your kin as possible would be ideal. Do you think they'd be willing to come to my office to speak with me? In private, of course."

"Probably not."

Warthin shakes his head. "I feared as much. People are as reluctant to talk about cancer as they are about tuberculosis or syphilis."

"My family's not reluctant—they're farmers."

"I see." Warthin smiles. "Well, I can assure you that I'll present things in the *simplest* way possible so there will be no misunderstanding."

Pauline corrects him. "I'm afraid it's *you* who doesn't understand. They're not ignorant. They're busy. It's hard work making sure the people of Ann Arbor have food to put on their tables."

The doctor colours, then says, "If they'll be as forthcoming with me as you are, then I'm more than willing to go to them. Consider me a census taker of sorts, only instead of counting acres and income, I'll be recording symptoms and such."

The statistics of death, Pauline thinks.

She was eight years old when the census takers came knocking on the doors of the farmhouses in Freedom Township. Her father had proudly welcomed them into their home and bragged about how his children were all in school, "English-only school, of course. Even the boys." The Swabian immigrants of the area were rightfully sensitive about their citizenship and their acceptance in society. There'd been plenty of talk among their Yankee neighbours about who did and didn't belong, and what constituted "good moral character." Many of her relatives had been anxious about being questioned by government officials about where they'd come from, who their parents were, if they could read and write.

"I'll need to go with you," she says.

"Pardon?"

"I'd like to go with you, to make introductions, explanations and so on."

"You'd be willing to do that?"

"Yes."

Returning to his notebook, Warthin writes in bold letters across the top of the page: FAMILY G, after the first initial of Pauline's surname. "In return for your family's cooperation, I'd like to issue an open invitation: anyone requiring medical attention may come to the University Hospital for care."

What he doesn't mention is his own desire to collect tissue samples from Pauline's kin, if and when they expire. As the new head of the university's pathology lab, he's eager to prove his worth. This is the sort of research that could become his life's work.

"Thank you, doctor," Pauline says, feeling hopeful about the arrangement. *With any luck,* she thinks, *it will keep us alive.*

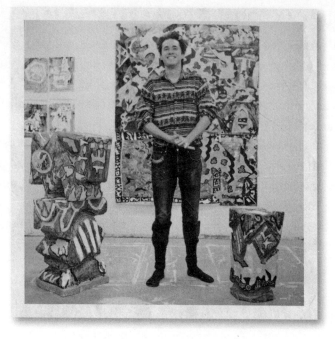

7.

The Seeds We Plant Today

Scots Bay, Nova Scotia, August 2017

In preparation for my talk with my eldest son, I begin retracing Pauline's steps, constructing a timeline of all our relatives who have died from cancer. Unlike my great-great aunt, though, I plan to document the positive milestones of their lives as well. I want my son to see that alongside pain and illness, there's been courage, joy and truth. I refuse to let this disease define us.

Maps, letters, journals, pedigree charts, death certificates, census records, city directories, newspaper clippings and personal anecdotes litter my desk. One by one, I pin bits and pieces of my research to the wall of my writing studio, transforming the room into a space that bears a striking resemblance to a fictional police precinct, complete with cluttered evidence board and half-empty cups of tepid coffee. I am the harried, obsessed investigator; and, as with any binge-worthy crime drama, there are mysteries to solve, love stories to be told and several ghosts waiting in the wings.

Spreading a roll of brown kraft paper on the floor, I get on my hands and knees to plot my family's history by the decade; beginning with 1830, when Pauline's grandfather (my great-great-great-grandfather) Johannes Haab arrived in America. Enticed by the promise of cheap, fertile land, he and his wife, Anna, left family and friends behind in Germany to immigrate to what was then Michigan Territory. Much to their dismay, the land was a forest that needed to be cleared if they wished to farm it. Determined not to fail, they built a homestead and barn, and began raising livestock and crops in order to provide for their growing family. Johannes Haab died from stomach cancer in the prime of his life, leaving Anna to run the farm and finish raising their children. Pauline's mother, Kathrina, was only ten when he passed.

My son is standing in my studio, staring at the length of kraft paper that's now attached to the wall. The timeline is over six feet long and I've only gotten to the summer of 1929.

"What do the red dots mean?" he asks.

"Those are deaths from cancer," I say.

"All of them?"

"Yes."

"Shit."

Seeing the family's litany of cancer deaths all in one place—name after name, decade after decade—is deeply unsettling. Even the colour of the paper tugs at my heart, reminiscent of the sewing patterns my mother, sister and I used to pluck from wide metal drawers at the fabric store before holiday parties and school dances. But that delicate tissue was the stuff of dreams, the dotted lines and black arrows point-ing the way to possibility and bliss.

"I don't want to nag," I tell him, even though that's what I'm doing. I've got a nephew not much older than him who's already tested positive for the gene. Thankfully, Lacie has just found out she's negative.

"You're not nagging, Mom. I'm going to get it done."

"When?"

"Soon."

"I'll help in any way I can, but you have to call the shots. Understand?"

"I do."

He's been home for the past two weeks, teaching at the summer arts camp where his sixteen-year-old brother is a counsellor. I'm incredibly proud of both of them, and of the life my husband and I have made in our corner of the world. It's been a lovely summer—bonfires at the beach, hikes in the woods, visits with family and friends from out of town. The perfect time to tackle my fears.

My son wraps his arms around me in a hug. "Love you, Mom." He's tall and lanky and soft-hearted, like my brothers.

"Love you too, kiddo."

That night I dream of my mother.

I'm walking in the woods alone when she appears out of nowhere, sitting on a moss-covered log in a thicket of hemlock and spruce. She looks solid, real, alive, but I know better than to touch her or be the first to speak. Ghosts have rules. I sit next to her and she smiles. She's healthy, tan, relaxed, younger than when she died. I'd guess she's about my age. Birds flit between the branches above our heads. I have no idea how long we sit there or what's going to happen next, but it's comforting all the same.

Eventually she says, "You have to go."

"But when I leave you'll disappear."

"I will?"

"I think so, yes."

"Don't worry, I'll be around again."

I believe her.

Before I go, she says one last thing, not out loud but in my thoughts: *all the flowers of all our tomorrows are in the seeds we plant today.*

It was her grandmother Tillie's favourite saying.

Mom repeated it to me throughout my childhood and well into my teens. I'd included it in my first novel as a secret message to her, knowing it would bring a smile to her face when she found it.

Sitting up in bed, I suddenly realize what it means. It's not just a simple gardener's saying passed on from grandmother to granddaughter, mother to daughter. It's an affirmation, an incantation to prevent life from kicking your ass. If you can believe that one seed you've sown, one deed you've done will flourish after you've gone, then you've beaten the curse. The towering hollyhocks and climbing roses that graced my great-grandmother's garden weren't just for show. They were beautiful, glorious fuck-yous to Death.

8.

Inheritance

Lebanon, Indiana, March 1983
Grade 9. My first year in high school. I'm doing well academically, but when it comes to social interaction I'm a loser, a failure, a nerd. I don't understand how popularity works. It seems to me that there's a shit-load of lying, cheating, drinking and blonde hair dye involved, and I don't know how to navigate any of it. Small-town friendship is a blood sport. Being fourteen sucks.

In their Lebanon High School yearbooks, my three siblings had been labelled "popular," "funny" and "sweet" by their classmates in '73, '74 and '80, respectively. When I graduate in 1986, the student body will vote me "most likely to live in her car."

Books serve as escape hatches to worlds where justice prevails, freaks win and outcasts are unlikely heroes. Poetry anthologies become my constant companions, large weighty volumes I can stick my nose into to avoid conversation, or clutch against my breasts as I walk the crowded, sweaty hallways of good old LHS. While pimple-faced boys riffle through my backpack for evidence that I'm "on the rag," I cling to secret messages Emily Dickinson has sent me through time. *"Hope" is the thing with feathers—/ That perches in the soul—*

I fall hard for the romantics: Byron, Keats, Shelley, Elizabeth Barrett Browning, Christina Rossetti. *There's blood between us, love, my love.* On one particularly angsty morning, I write in the back of my English Lit. notebook: *If any man ever recites "She Walks in Beauty" to me (from memory), my heart is his.*

My mom makes a habit of reminding me that high school is just a stepping stone to university. "You'll find your tribe there, I'm sure of it."

Four years feels like an eternity.

When I'm not reading I'm practicing piano, playing French horn or singing. Music gives me a way of being in the world without feeling completely awkward and lost. I join concert band and chorus. I ace try-outs for show choir because my grandmother Alice knows all the jazz standards on the audition list and insists on singing them with me until I've got them by heart. "After You've Gone." "Look for the Silver Lining." "Till We Meet Again."

"Everyone said my sister Grace was the musical one, but I was in just as many mus-i-cales as she was. I even sang with the Chautauqua Players that came round in the summer. They asked me to go with them on the road, but my parents wouldn't allow it."

"How old were you?"

"Old enough to know better, according to my mother," Alice says with a laugh. Then she clutches her side and winces.

"You all right?"

"Just my diverticulitis acting up," she says, motioning to the half-empty bowl of popcorn on the coffee table between us. "Guess I had more than I should."

We'd taken turns scooping handfuls of popcorn into our mouths while watching Indiana play Kentucky in the NCAA basketball tournament. I knew she wasn't supposed to eat it, but she'd sworn to me "a little won't hurt." By the time Bobby Knight (who, according to Alice, had his head up his ass) had failed to bring the Hoosiers to victory in the Sweet 16, she was doubly sore.

"I'll go get Mom," I say, worried that Alice's pain was about to turn into a trip to the hospital.

"No," she says, brushing me off. "It'll work itself out. It's not like I have much plumbing left in there for it to matter anyway."

I pick up the bowl and head for the trailer's kitchenette. I figure I'd better put temptation out of reach. It's a short trip from the living room, only a few steps, but I take care not to disturb Alice's latest "project" along the way.

She's been labelling every object she owns according to "who'll get it when I die." Strips of yellow legal pad are now pinned, taped, stapled and thumbtacked to needlepoint pillows, picture frames, teacup handles and chair legs, each one bearing an initial for my uncle, aunt and mother. I have trouble finding a place for the greasy popcorn bowl in the kitchen. Alice's tiny table is cluttered with unassigned bits of paper and antique guidebooks. My grampy's enormous volume of *Audubon's Birds of America* sits askew on a chair next to the windowsill where his binoculars have been gathering dust for the past three years.

Alice is still insisting she wants to die. She says it's because she misses my grandfather, but I wonder if that's true. When he was alive, all I ever saw them do was say snide things to each other and pretend not to hear them. It didn't look like love to me. Yet Alice insisted that once upon a time James H. Mackintosh was "witty, charming, a bit of a joker," a boy from the eastern seaboard who loved nature and art, and didn't quite know how to handle spending the rest of his life landlocked. He and Alice ran a kennel together on the east side of Indianapolis where they boarded dogs and raised American Kennel Club cocker spaniels. He was always looking for the pick of the litter to bring them best in show. By the time I came around, he was broke and bitter. My mom said that's what happens when a Scotsman is born on St. Patrick's Day. My dad said it was because he got caught not paying his taxes.

I set the bowl next to the sink and go back to the living room. Alice is slumped in her chair with her head in her hands.

"Are you having more pain?" I ask. "Is there anything I can do?"

She looks at me with tears streaming down her face. "I've been terrible to your mother."

I grab a tissue and hand it to her. I've never heard her admit it. "It'll be all right," I tell her. "She loves you."

"I wouldn't blame her if she didn't."

I sit next to Alice in silence. I don't know what to say.

She cries harder. "I did an awful thing . . ."

I have no idea what she's talking about. My mom hasn't mentioned any new arguments between them, hasn't complained more than usual to my dad. "What did you do?" I ask.

"It was back when she was your age. I'm sure she must've told you."

"I'm sure she didn't."

Alice wipes her eyes, blows her nose, takes a sip of cold coffee. The mug clatters on the table as she sets it down. "I sold her away . . . to another family."

This is the first I've heard of it. I'm shocked, confused, angry. "Why would you do that?"

Getting up from her chair Alice heads towards her bedroom. "I need to lie down."

I follow after her. "Why would you sell my mother?"

She lies on her bed, turns her back to me and refuses to answer.

Sitting on the edge of the bed in my parents' room, I wait for my mother. I run my hand across her pink satin pillowcase. I remove the lid from the bottle of Youth-Dew on her vanity and take a sniff. Patchouli. Rose. Jasmine. Moss. Spices. This is where I go when I need to talk to her, in private.

She walks in, shuts the door and sits next to me. "What's this all about, sweetheart?" She loops my hair behind my ear. She knows I'm upset.

There's no easy way to tell her about Alice's confession so I simply come out with it. "Alice says she sold you, when you were a girl."

My mother takes a deep breath. "I see."

"Is it true?"

"This stays between you and me."

"Okay."

"Your grampy was out of work, and he and your grandmother couldn't make ends meet. Your uncle was still a boy and your aunt was just a baby. There was a family in town who said they'd take me in if I helped out around the house, did some cooking and cleaning."

She's trying to make it sound reasonable. "So you went to live with strangers?" I can't imagine it.

"I didn't have a choice. My clothes were getting too small and we didn't have money to buy new ones. I'd already made my winter coat last an extra winter by ripping the lining in the sleeves so they'd cover my wrists. It was summer, so I was out of school. I was the oldest. My mother said I had to do it."

"How old were you?"

"Thirteen."

I feel like I'm going to be sick. "Were they nice to you, at least?"

"I suppose. What they really wanted was a maid and what they got was a child. I didn't know what I was doing. Eventually they told me to go home because I didn't suit their needs. I was ashamed and scared so I hitched a ride on a hay truck to my grandma Tillie's."

"How far was it to her place?"

"About thirty miles."

I'm afraid to ask more questions, but I need to know the rest of the story. "What did your grandmother say?"

"Not much, which was probably for the best. She took me in for the rest of the summer. I helped out at the drugstore my grandfather ran in Saline, and at home in Tillie's kitchen. That's when I learned to cook and sew my own clothes."

It's where she learned to be a mother.

"And you went home after that? Back to your parents'?"

"I did. I missed my little brother and baby sister. And even though Alice had sent me away, I still loved her."

I hug my mom and don't let go.

She cries on my shoulder.

For the first time in my life I understand her.

9.

Alterations

Ann Arbor, Michigan, 1898

A young bride stands on a low wooden stool, her new satin shoes creaking as she nervously shifts her weight from side to side.

"Hold still, please," Pauline directs. "I need to check the hem."

The bride does as she's told.

Her mother and her future mother-in-law circle her, looking for imperfections. The bride's mother stares at the dress. The groom's mother, at the bride. Pauline tries her best to hold the young woman's attention.

"Chin up, shoulders back," she says, then steps forward and slips a pin into the seam at the left shoulder of the dress. The girl's posture is askew, owing to a slight but permanent tilt in her left hip. If the shoulder of the dress isn't corrected, the entire line of the gown will reveal the defect. Addressing the problem will mean taking apart the sleeve and bodice.

Upon completing her inspection of the bride, the groom's mother addresses the mother of the bride. "Did you hear that Mrs. Blake's daughter-in-law is expecting, *again?*"

"Sadly, yes," the woman replies. "Although I can't say it surprises me. The girl was raised in a home simply overflowing with children. It's in her blood."

The bride sucks in her belly and holds her breath, anticipating the inevitable.

She's next, Pauline thinks. She casts no judgment on the matter, just makes allowances as necessary.

"The girl *is* terribly romantic-looking, isn't she?" the groom's mother quips.

The bride's mother gives a knowing laugh. "Precisely. The Germans in this town certainly take after the rabbits they're so fond of eating."

Both these women are members of the Ladies' Aid Society, the Women's League, and the Woman's Christian Temperance Union. Their husbands are professors at the university. They believe in social purity and good breeding.

Pauline, being rather romantic-looking herself, ignores them and carries on with her work. She could easily get revenge by not properly looking after the alterations to the girl's dress, but she's got nothing against the bride. The girl has kind eyes and is a good listener, which makes Pauline hopeful that she'll turn out to be different from the woman who raised her.

Speech is silver, but silence is golden.

After settling accounts with the bride's mother, Pauline gathers her things and heads to the university hospital to visit her cousin Rosa, who'd been admitted two weeks earlier. Pauline had asked Tillie to join her, but her sister had refused. "I don't think I can bear it," she'd said.

Pauline doesn't know if she can either, but she feels she must go. She's the reason Rosa was there in the first place.

Rosa had fallen ill in the same terrible way so many other women in the family had before her. Her monthly bleeding grew heavy and the horrible pain that accompanied it eventually stayed and never left. Tired, pale and weak, she could barely bring herself to get out of bed.

She lived several hours to the north of Ann Arbor, but she'd heard through the family grapevine that Pauline and Dr. Warthin had been making the rounds of the old homesteads in Washtenaw County. She'd heard talk of talented doctors, free hospital visits, maybe even a cure. Anxious, Rosa had decided to make the trek south, thinking there must be something the doctors at the university could do to help her. It was a full day's journey by train.

The doctors took her medical history, ran a series of tests, and diagnosed her with cancer of the uterus. They advised her that a hysterectomy was her only chance for survival. She agreed to the operation.

She was only forty-two. She had a husband and three daughters. She loved them fiercely, dearly. She wasn't ready to die.

By the time Pauline arrives at the hospital, Rosa has died from a post-operative infection: toxemia.

Stricken with grief, Pauline walks to Forest Hill to be alone with her thoughts. It's late May and the cemetery is in full bloom. Bridal wreath bushes burst with cascades of white blossoms along the pathway. Crabapple petals flutter in the air. *Rosa will never see such beauty again.*

Pauline can't help but wonder if her cousin would've been better off staying at home. *She would've had more time with her daughters. Died peacefully in her own bed, on her own terms.* It's been nearly three years since she'd first confessed her family's woes to Dr. Warthin, and Pauline's not sure anything good has come from it.

The pathologist is precise, dogmatic, even obsessed. For the most part, she admires him—his attitude, in many ways, is similar to how she is when it comes to work—but the more time she spends with him the more she begins to question his approach. In his quest for every detail, he is pushy during the interview process, pressing for information that's personal, intimate and painful to recall. Her relatives, in turn, have become reluctant to share anything with him at all.

"A little restraint would go a long way towards gaining their trust," she tells him. "I suggest you try using some."

"You sound like my colleagues."

"Maybe your colleagues have a point."

"Let them swear at me in the laboratory, so long as they swear by my methods in their practice."

His arrogance is deafening. "My relatives are not your colleagues, and this is no laboratory. You are a guest in our lives."

Mrs. Rosa Baessler Rodgers died Tuesday from the result of an operation, aged 42 years. Mrs. Rodgers was a daughter of the late Peter Baessler, of Ann Arbor town, and has lived in the northern part of the state for several years past. The funeral services will be held at the old

Baessler homestead and the remains will be interred in the Bethlehem Cemetery in Scio.

The sparse, half-true obituary comes nowhere close to describing Rosa's plight or the family's sadness, helplessness and shame. It doesn't name the husband and daughters she left behind. Nor does it mention her mother, Rosina, who'd met the same fate. Each death from cancer in the family not only weighs on Pauline's heart as a terrible loss, but also serves as proof that they are broken, beyond repair.

When she tries to talk about this with Warthin, he says, "Your cousin's time here wasn't for nothing. Her life wasn't lived in vain." To him, Rosa represents a victory. Her presence in the university hospital had meant he'd been able to gain a first-hand account of the disease rather than rely on second-hand memories. What's more, he'd finally been able to acquire tissue samples from a member of Family G. Being able to wed histology with the stories and case histories he's been gathering makes him feel as if he's uncovered an important clue.

Pauline says, "Our loss is your gain."

Warthin frowns. The dressmaker has hit a nerve. "Please don't think of it that way."

He'd examined Rosa's tissue sample every day since her death, staring at it under his microscope, memorizing its whorls, loops, spots and curves. It's only natural for him to long for more specimens, more evidence. But that, of course, only comes at great cost. "Don't mistake my attitude for indifference, Miss Gross. I'm confident my research will benefit you and your family and perhaps the entire world some day."

"One can only hope," Pauline says.

10.

Previvor

Port Williams, Nova Scotia, October 2017

I have an eleven o'clock appointment with my internist, Dr. Stern. He's retiring next month, so this will be our last meeting as patient and doctor. It feels strange to think of it. He's been with me since the start of my journey with Lynch syndrome.

"How are you feeling?" he asks, as he escorts me into his office. "Everything all right?"

"I'm doing well, thanks."

I settle into a chair. He sits behind his desk.

"No problems with your bowel or gut? No significant changes?"

"Nope. It's all good."

His office windows look across the dykes that run along the Cornwallis River. The landscape is awash with the hazy sunlight of early autumn, every rock, tree and blade of grass bathed with dusky gold. His desk is positioned so he's got the best view.

I don't resent it. He's a serious birder like my grampy was, always on the lookout for his next "lifer," the latest bird he's never seen.

One of the few pleasant memories I have of my grandfather is of sitting with a Peterson's field guide in my lap and a wooden birdcall strung around my neck as he instructed me on the finer points of bird watching. *Warblers can be tricky to tell apart, especially in the fall. The flighty, nervous buggers never sit still.* I like to think that Dr. Stern's passion for birding gives him an edge when it comes to catching suspicious-looking tumours in the gut.

"I guess I should congratulate you on your retirement," I say. "But I have to admit, I'm sad you're leaving."

"I'm not all that happy about it either. I'm not sure I'm ready to go."

That surprises me. I'd imagined that a career of sticking a scope where the sun don't shine might leave a person eager to call it quits. "Why not?"

"I'll miss the camaraderie at the hospital and getting together with colleagues to exchange ideas."

"I guess I'd miss that too."

"It's not the same as it once was, though. Hospital staff are incredibly busy, less inclined to stop for lengthy discussions."

Countless breakthroughs in medical research have occurred because of chance meetings, random discussions and serendipitous turns. Lives have been saved. If there's no room in a physician's daily life for consultation with their peers, then there's probably scant time for proper patient care as well. This is the current state of our medical system and it scares me. I've been fortunate to have this bespectacled, sensible Brit looking after me all these years. I don't know who I'll get next. "I'm going to miss having you in my corner."

In 2002, I'd handed my family doctor a pile of medical literature along with my genetic test results. He'd listened intently as I'd talked him through the ins and outs of Lynch syndrome, then he'd sent me a list of specialists to shepherd me through the long series of recommended annual tests and screenings. Dr. Stern had been first on the list.

"I see you're positive for the MSH2 mutation," he'd said, looking up from my file. "Are you aware that the risk for colorectal cancer with that particular Lynch syndrome gene is quite high? The chance you'll develop it is around 85 percent, and the average age of onset is forty-six."

"I'm aware," I'd said. "You don't need to convince me to get a colonoscopy." Physically, I felt fine, but I was anxious to get my first scope. I knew all too well that Lynch syndrome colon cancers are hard to detect. They present with raised, flat-headed tumours instead of polyps, and in my family's case, usually at the far end of the colon near the cecum. The tumours grow incredibly fast and are prone to spread. If undetected, they can kill you in a matter of months.

"It says here you're an unaffected carrier. So you've never had cancer?"

"No, I haven't."

"Then how did you come to be tested for Lynch syndrome? It's usually not considered until after a patient has been diagnosed with cancer."

I gave him the short version of my immediate family's medical history. "I can go further back if you like. Researchers have been studying my family since 1895."

"*Eighteen* ninety-five?" I could tell he thought he'd misheard me.

"I wrote a radio documentary about it that aired a couple of months ago on the CBC. You can listen to it online. There's an interview with Dr. Lynch in it as well."

"*The* Dr. Lynch?"

"Yes. Henry's known my family since before I was born."

"Well, isn't that something." Stern was staring at me as if I were a rare bird who'd been blown off course and landed in his office.

I was just thankful to be talking to someone outside my family who knew what Lynch syndrome was.

Making a note in my file he'd said, "I recommend that you have annual colonoscopies. Have you ever had one before?"

"No."

"I'll schedule one for you as soon as possible."

Colonoscopy number fifteen was two days after the Women's March of 2017. January 21, I'd marched. January 22, I'd purged. January 23, I'd gone to the hospital for what had become an annual ritual.

The nurse who had led me into the room for my scope was someone I'd never met. "This is Dr. Stern," she'd announced. "He'll be the one performing your procedure."

"No need for introductions," I'd said, climbing up on the examination bed. "We're old friends."

"How'd the prep go?" Dr. Stern asked in greeting.

"Squeaky clean."

"Let's have a look then, shall we?"

One nurse prepped my arm for light sedation while another attached a heart monitor to the end of my finger. I made small talk with Dr. Stern while we waited for the drugs to kick in. "Any recent bird sightings of note?"

"I had over a hundred waxwings in my yard last week—cedar and bohemian. They stripped my crabapple trees bare of any fruit still hanging."

"They did the same at my place. The pretty piggies' beaks were covered with mushy fruit by the time they were done."

He checked the scope then adjusted the monitor he'd be watching during the procedure. "I gave Liz your latest novel for Christmas. She really enjoyed it. She's hoping you might have time to visit her reading group?"

"Sure." I was more than happy to make time for his lovely wife. "Have her email me so we can make arrangements."

"Thanks, I will." Scope in hand, Dr. Stern brought our chitchat to an end. "Are we ready?"

I gave him a slightly woozy thumbs-up.

It was difficult not to be nervous. In addition to wanting a clear, cancer-free colonoscopy, I needed to stay somewhat alert so I could follow any instructions he had for me as we went along. This meant I'd feel some pain. I have the misfortune of being born with a tortuous colon, complete with extra hairpin twists and turns. This makes colonoscopies difficult to perform.

Facing the monitor, I watched as Dr. Stern went about his business. My gut looked healthy and clean. When I wasn't staring at my intestines, I was checking out a small square in the upper left corner of the screen. Dr. Stern had gotten a new program that was mapping a virtual image of my colon. He wasn't kidding when he'd said it was a tricky twisted thing.

"Hold your breath," one of the nurses instructed as Dr. Stern prepared to manoeuvre past a sharp turn.

I let out a groan. The last couple of turns on the way to my cecum are always the hardest.

"All right now, you can breathe."

It wasn't easy for any of us, but through concentration and team effort, we'd eventually reached the end. As Dr. Stern backed the scope out he declared, "It's all good." I'd been awarded my golden ticket for another year.

In the recovery room I texted my husband, sons, brothers and sister: "Pink, smooth and clear!"

A string of smiling poo emojis appeared on my screen.

"Woohoo!"

"Yay sis!"

"Way to go, Mom!"

Lynch syndrome families are wonderfully weird.

Now, as I sit across from Dr. Stern, I can't believe we're about to say goodbye. "Got any farewell advice for me?" I ask.

"Are you still taking aspirin?"

"Three hundred and twenty-five milligrams per day."

He'd read a medical study stating there was evidence that Lynch syndrome patients who take aspirin on a daily basis have a lower risk of developing colorectal cancer. To date, it'd been the only proactive step (aside from prophylactic surgeries) that I could take to prevent a Lynch syndrome cancer. Being fit and eating healthy made me feel good, but it didn't make a bit of difference to my mutation. The aspirin wasn't a sure thing, but we'd agreed it was worth a try.

"Anything else?" I ask.

"Yes, but I think you already know what it is."

My heart fills with dread as I ready myself for what he's about to say. We've had the same conversation several times over in the past few years. "I can guess."

"Well, my opinion hasn't changed. Your tortuous colon makes your scopes painful and difficult to complete. Under those circumstances, it's quite possible something could be missed. Because of this,

I think you should have a colectomy. Your odds of getting colon cancer only get worse as you get older. Having the surgery while you're young and healthy can save you from a lot of suffering."

I understand why he feels the need to repeat himself, but that doesn't make it any easier to take. What he's asking me to do is have my entire colon preemptively removed. Logically it makes sense, but emotionally I have a hell of a time wrapping my head around it. Yanking out five feet of intestines doesn't come without risks, even if you're in perfect health. I've seen the best and worst of it. My oldest brother's cancer was caught early enough that he didn't require chemo, so all he had to worry about was recovering from the surgery. (No small feat.) He worked like hell to teach his body how to function properly again, and then went on to compete in a few triathlons in his mid-fifties. My mom wasn't so lucky. Surgery and two rounds of chemo after her second bout of colon cancer had left her body weak and fragile. It'd been more than she could take.

Over the years Dr. Stern had referred me to several different surgeons for consultation. I'd diligently met with each one and listened to their take on how they'd handle the operation. It's a surgery that's almost exclusively performed on those who already have cancer. Rarely, if ever, is it done as a preemptive strike. To a one, the surgeons had all agreed it was a highly unusual step, even for someone with Lynch syndrome, but also worth serious consideration given my situation. Dr. Stern had patiently followed up after each appointment, the dutiful matchmaker hoping I'd like one of the surgeons well enough to finally take the leap.

"So when are you going to get the surgery?" he asks. This last time he's going all in.

"I've been thinking fifty might be the right time."

He checks the birth date on my file. "So this next year then, 2018?"

I balk. "Maybe."

"What's keeping you from it?"

"I've got deadlines, and some travelling I'd like to do." I'll give any excuse rather than admit I'm scared out of my wits.

Twirling a pen between his fingers he says, "I want you to be able to do *all* the things you want to do."

"I need to find the right time. It's not just the surgery, but the recovery too."

"Your recovery will be much harder if you've got cancer to contend with."

He knows that's how my mother died.

A voice screams in my head: *If it ain't broke, don't fix it.*

I've already had one prophylactic surgery, a hysterectomy two days before my forty-fifth birthday, to ward off the gynecological cancers related to Lynch syndrome. It took me over a decade to decide to do it. Such choices are emotionally taxing and complex, yet part and parcel of carrying a genetic mutation that predisposes you to cancer, of being a "previvor."

My goal is to hold that title for as long as possible.

AMI MCKAY
previvor

If I had such cards made today, how many would I order? Five hundred? A thousand? A lifetime supply?

Dr. Stern closes my file. He's said his piece.

He meets my eyes. "I'm sorry for all those dreadful colonoscopies."

"I'm sorry about my kinky colon," I reply, then stand. "I'm truly grateful for all your attention and care. You've given me and my family much-needed peace of mind."

Dr. Stern comes around from behind his desk and gives me a hug. "Take care of yourself, Ami."

His warmth catches me off guard. I think of the choices I still need to make, of my dear husband and our two sons, of all the things I haven't done. "I will," I say. "I promise."

II.

The Inmost Part of You

Lebanon, Indiana, 1984

My mom grabs a tube of lipstick from her makeup drawer in the bathroom—dusky rose to match her dress. She spritzes her upswept do with hairspray, lines her arched brows, swipes her cheeks with blush. The dress she's wearing is slightly off the shoulder, with dolman sleeves and a flowing skirt. It's elegant, understated, a bit flirtatious.

"Presentable?" she asks, as we stand together in front of the mirror.

"You look great, Mom," I answer, awed by her ability to go from jeans and a sweatshirt to pure glamour in a matter of minutes.

"There's a container of beef stroganoff on the kitchen counter for your supper. All you have to do is boil some noodles and heat up the sauce."

She's going dancing with Dad. There's a band playing down at the Legion ("jazz standards and oldies instead of that awful country rock"). They're headed out to dinner before they hit the dance floor.

Dad grabs Mom by the hand, whisks her down the hall and into the living room. Loose change jangles in his pocket as he spins her around. "Would you look at your mom?" he asks with a grin. "Isn't she the prettiest gal you've ever seen?"

I smile and nod. He's been doing this same adorable shtick for as long as I can remember. It doesn't matter if Mom is in her best dress or walking around the house with curlers in her hair. He'll take any opportunity he gets to tell the world how spectacular he thinks she is. They've been married thirty years but still act like newlyweds.

"I've said it before and I'll say it again," he says, bending Mom in a deep dip, "I'd be nothing but a lousy bum if she hadn't married me. Your mother saved my life."

"We saved each other," my mother corrects.

I'd grown up watching them dance together, spinning records one after another on their old hi-fi. Tony Bennett, Ella Fitzgerald, Herb Alpert & the Tijuana Brass. They'd started their vinyl collection when they were first married, back when Dad was still in the navy and stationed at Moffett Field in California after the Korean War. They didn't have much income, so they'd spent their "mad money" each week to buy a new record or two, then stayed home and played gin rummy.

"Don't have any wild parties while we're gone," Dad jokes as he helps Mom with her coat.

"It's not me you have to worry about," I tell him. "It's Alice. She's the wild one."

Dad laughs.

Mom doesn't.

Alice has taken to being strategically neglectful, of her house, her body, her health, especially whenever my mom has something going on. I can tell Mom's nervous about tonight.

Pausing at the door, Dad says, "I told your grandmother we'd be going out and that you'd be here alone. You don't have to go over there, but you might give her a call before it gets too late, let her know you're okay?" He thinks Alice will be less prone to act up if she feels she's needed.

"No problem, Dad. I'll do it."

Dad gives me a wink as he picks Mom up and sweeps her down the steps.

Bursting into giggles she calls, "Don't wait up!"

I consider the stroganoff then make a PB&J instead. I've got an English paper due tomorrow on the nature of madness in *Hamlet*.

Setting my boom box at the end of my bed, I slide Prince and the Revolution's *Purple Rain* into the tape deck and hit play. Cranking the volume, I cut loose to "Let's Go Crazy." Normally I have to listen to the album on headphones (Mom would freak if she heard the lyrics to "Dear Nikki") so it's a rush to blare it through the house. Prince is complex, dramatic, sexy, a complete genius. He's got more in common with Shakespeare than not.

To be, or not to be—that is the question;

"Take Me with U." "The Beautiful Ones." "Computer Blue."

> *to die: to sleep*
> *No more, and by a sleep to say we end*
> *The heartache and the thousand natural shocks*
> *That flesh is heir to: 'tis a consummation*
> *Devoutly to be wished—To die: to sleep—*

"Darling Nikki." "When Doves Cry." "I Would Die 4 U."

> *To sleep, perchance to dream—ay, there's the rub,*
> *For in that sleep of death what dreams may come,*
> *When we have shuffled off this mortal coil,*
> *Must give us pause: there's the respect*
> *That makes calamity of so long life.*

Existential crisis. Family baggage. Seduction.

The phone rings. It's Alice. Her voice is shaky. "Come quick," she says, then hangs up.

I run next door and find her lying in bed. Her face is pale and her belly's bloated, hard as a rock. Her lips and tongue are coated in something white and chalky.

"I thought I'd have a glass of Bromo-Seltzer before bed," she whispers, "but something's not right." She clutches her stomach and groans.

There's a spoon and an empty glass on her nightstand alongside a jar with no label, half-full of white powder. The jar's lid is rusty and loose. I recognize the container as one that usually sits on the counter next to her washing machine. I pray it's not the powdered bleach she likes to use on her sheets. *Stay calm,* I think. *Don't panic.* I reach for the phone to dial for help.

Alice waves my hand away. "I already called for an ambulance."

Sirens scream up the driveway. Flashing lights flood through the windows.

I open the door for a pair of paramedics and point to Alice's room. "She said she took Bromo, but I'm pretty sure that's not what it was." I hand over the jar.

They rush to Alice's side and immediately start assessing her condition. They shine a light in her eyes, ask her name, take her blood pressure.

One of the paramedics turns to me. "Is she on any medication?"

"She takes a lot of different drugs. I don't know the names."

Alice does. "Tagamet for my hiatal hernia, Percocet for pain . . ."

While she rattles off the rest of her meds, I call the Legion and ask for my dad.

"Jesus," he says. "Is she all right?"

"I'm not sure."

One of the paramedics says calmly to Alice, "We need to take you to the hospital to pump your stomach, just in case."

I relay the information to Dad while my grandmother is loaded onto a stretcher.

"You can ride along with us," the tech says. "Tell your parents we'll meet them there."

"Did you hear that, Dad?"

"Roger that, kiddo. See you soon."

A couple hours later, Alice is propped up in a hospital bed and holding court with the nursing staff. She looks strangely angelic in the low fluorescent light, satisfied and calm after all this attention.

I sit by her side while Mom and Dad stand by the door, waiting for an update from the doctor.

Turning to me, Alice says, "See if one of the nurses can't find a hand mirror? I must look a fright."

Come, come, and sit you down. You shall not budge.
You go not till I set you up a glass
Where you may see the inmost part of you.

The doctor arrives and tells my parents, "We'll be keeping her overnight, for observation."

Dad squeezes Mom's hand.

Taking Mom aside, the doctor hands her the jar. "The nearest we can tell is that it's some sort of detergent."

Mom opens the jar and takes a sniff. "Borax," she says.

"The good news is she was never in any real danger."

Mom's face freezes in a strained smile. "Thank heavens for that."

"Come here," Alice motions to me, holding out her hand.

I do as she says.

"This is my granddaughter," she tells the doctor. "She came running as soon as I called. I don't know what I'd do without her." She's pointedly staring across the room at my mom.

Dad puts a stop to it. "How about we get out of here and let you get some rest, Alice?"

Mom is already at the door.

"Sally," Alice calls to her. "Aren't you going to say goodnight?"

But look, amazement on thy mother sits.
O, step between her and her fighting soul.
Conceit in weakest bodies strongest works.
Speak to her, Hamlet.

Mom stops and goes to Alice and kisses her forehead. "Be good, Mother. I'll see you tomorrow."

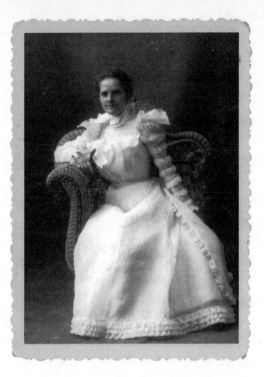

12

In Their Joys and in Their Sorrows

Ann Arbor, Michigan, 1900

Dressed in a beautiful gown trimmed with delicate ruffles and hand-made lace, Tillie sits in a wicker photographer's chair. Her wedding is only a few days away. She stares into the camera, her poise saying as much about the gown as it does the bride-to-be. Leaning on her elbow, she gracefully extends her other arm. She means to show off the exquisite sleeve of her dress along with her sister's craftsmanship and talent. From wrist to shoulder, the Mamaluke sleeves are shirred and pouffed no less than eight times. Three tiers of pin-tucked ruffles grace the hem of the dress. Its high-boned collar, square yoke and pigeon chest are triumphs of the latest style. It's Pauline's greatest work to date.

Circling around her sister, Pauline inspects the dress's neck, sleeves, waist, hem. Spotting a wayward crease, she gently tugs at the bottom of the skirt.

"Stop fussing," Tillie says. "You're making me nervous."

Taking a pin from a cushion that's tied to her wrist, Pauline secures a small section of the dress's hem to Tillie's petticoat. The wrinkle disappears. "I never met a bride who wasn't."

The photographer clears his throat, checks his watch, but Pauline will not be hurried. Seeing her sister in her wedding dress, sunlight streaming through the windows and across her dear face is a dream come true. She'll take all the time she needs. The photographer will have to wait.

All morning she's had visions of herself and Tillie as girls—laughing, running through the barnyard, unkempt braids slapping their backs. They'd been best friends, inseparable. Soon all that will change.

Stepping back, she finally nods. "She's ready."

The photographer adjusts the position of his camera on its tripod and prepares to remove the cover from the lens. "All right, miss," he says. "Don't blink."

Tillie stares at him serenely.

Pauline takes a handkerchief from her pocket and wipes a tear from her eye.

"Thank you, miss," the photographer says. "That's perfect."

Yes, Pauline thinks. *She is.*

The time the two sisters spend together in the days before the wedding is joyful yet bittersweet. There is their imminent parting to consider as well as the topsy-turvy nature of a youngest daughter marrying before her older sister. Their age difference isn't vast, but for the longest time everyone in the family had been placing bets on when Pauline would pair off with the dashing professor from the university.

Everyone except Pauline.

It wasn't like that. It never had been.

Such speculation had been laid to rest in early summer, when Aldred Warthin had married Katherine Angell, a smart young physician from Chicago. She was a good match for the stubborn, brusque bachelor. It was common knowledge that she'd pointedly turned him down at least once before she'd finally said yes.

"He wasn't good enough for you," Tillie had insisted. "You deserve a man who will treat you like a queen." She'd just become engaged to O.C. Wheeler, a lanky young pharmacist from Ann Arbor, with striking blue eyes and Yankee blood. They were over-the-moon in love. It was the start of a new century, the era of "anything is possible" in the American Midwest. O.C. was twenty-seven, Tillie twenty-three. "You'll find your match someday soon, Pauline, I'm sure of it."

Pauline didn't have the heart to tell her sister that she had no intention of getting married. *Why look for true love when you know your life is going to be cut short?* In addition to her personal convictions, Dr. Warthin had strongly suggested that someone with her family history should think long and hard before marrying and having children. He'd likened her family's bloodline to inferior stock, "the breeding of which results in sub-par offspring. As the daughter of a farmer, I'm sure you understand."

"Yes," she'd replied. " I do."

She'd never question her sister's right to happiness, or anyone else's in the family, but as far as she was concerned, the matter was settled.

Mr and Mrs Johann Frederick Gross,

announce the marriage of their daughter,

MATILDA ANNE

to

MR. OSCAR CHARLES WHEELER

On Thursday, the fourth of October,

nineteen hundred,

At the St. Thomas Lutheran Church

Freedom Township, Michigan

On a clear evening in early autumn, Tillie walks down the aisle of the St. Thomas Lutheran Church. It's the same small chapel where she and her siblings were baptized, the same modest sanctuary with arched windows and wooden pews in which she sat every Sunday throughout her childhood, reciting scripture and singing hymns in German. Women on the left, men on the right.

Bless them in their work and their companionship; in their sleeping and their waking; in their joys and in their sorrows; in their life and in their death.

Five months later, Tillie confesses to Pauline that she's pregnant. Holding her skirt taut against her belly, she turns in profile. "You see it, right?"

"I do," Pauline replies.

"What's wrong?" Tillie asks. "You're not smiling. Aren't you glad for me?"

Holding out her hand, Pauline motions for her sister to sit. "There's something I need to tell you. I thought it best I do it in person."

Tillie takes a seat. "What is it?" she asks, reaching for Pauline's hand.

"Mama's sick."

"Like Rosa?"

"Yes. I'm leaving Ann Arbor to help out at home."

Tillie's brow knots. "Why isn't Mama coming here to the hospital? Surely your Dr. Warthin has figured something out by now. Maybe the surgery they performed on Rosa will work this time around?"

Pauline had tried to make that same case with their mother and failed. Her mother would have none of it, saying, "Ann Arbor is dirty and crowded, and so is your professor's hospital."

"But Mama . . . the longer you wait—"

"Why do you suppose the doctors there are always asking us questions? It's because *we* know things *they* don't. When it's my time, I'll say my goodbyes at home. Not with strangers in the room like Rosa did."

Pauline tells her sister, "Mama doesn't trust the doctors at the university. She's been keeping her illness a secret, and now she's too far gone."

"Is there anything I can do? Any way I can help?"

"You can take care of yourself and the wee one."

Pauline trades her quiet room at the boarding house for her family's bustling homestead. Her eldest brother, Samuel, still lives at home and runs the farm alongside their father. Her three youngest brothers are still in school: Albert, sixteen; Elmer, eleven; and Rudolph, nine. It's a struggle to keep the boys in line.

It's even more of a task to convince her mother that she should take on the household chores. "Please, Mama, you must let me help."

"I've spent the last thirty years keeping my husband and children fed, clothed, loved and safe. I'm not about to stop now." There's anger in her voice, and frustration in every move she makes as her body grows weaker. "I thought the curse would pass us by." She's only fifty-five.

Day after day to the very end, Pauline chases after her mother with comfort and love.

On a bright afternoon in early fall, shortly after Tillie's first wedding anniversary, Kathrina Gross is laid to rest in the cemetery adjacent to St. Thomas Church. With her goes the dream that her own house might go untouched.

KATHRINA GROSS

Geb. 17 Sept 1847

Gest. 8 Okt 1901

PHIL. 1:23 *For I am in a strait betwixt two, having a desire to depart, and to be with Christ; which is far better.*

13.

Sehnsucht

Scots Bay, Nova Scotia, October 2017

Birth, life, death.

The cycle plays out in every family, in every corner of the world *ad infinitum*. We take joy in new beginnings, celebrate milestones, and grieve our losses—especially when the parting comes too soon. We sing, dance, love, weep—miraculous and commonplace; surprising yet inevitable.

Over a century after my great-great-grandmother's passing, her death stops me cold. Beyond the blood ties between us, I feel connected to Kathrina by who I am at this moment in my life: a mother, a wife, a woman of middle age. What will I do if/when cancer finds me?

Sehnsucht is a German word defined as an intense longing for something that is unknown and incomplete. It's what I feel when I think of Kathrina, who, by her choices, cleared the path for my existence. The unfairness of her death makes me heartsick. It also gives me cause to shun despair. Each morning she woke with a choice to either fear death or dance with it. She chose to dance.

I chase after her children, hoping to sort the details of their lives. *What happened to them? Where did they go? What did they do after their mother died?* I have stories Alice and my mother told me when I was young but it's not enough. It never will be.

There's no one left for me to ask all the questions I have nagging in my brain, so I rely on other sources—county record offices, local history museums, genealogical societies. Praise-be for the women who wrote society columns in small-town newspapers during the early twentieth century. Their obsession with bridal showers, garden parties and ladies' teas provides tantalizing insight into the lives of my ancestors.

Turning to Kathrina's death certificate first, I study the document line by line. I can see why Dr. Warthin made a practice of collecting them. They provide important data about the deceased: age, cause of death, contributing factors and so on, along with the names of attending doctors, coroners and undertakers—men he'd eagerly sought out in hopes they'd shed new light on each case.

My takeaways are slightly different than his. I immediately notice that on this document Kathrina is referred to by her Americanized name, "Catherine," and her father is listed as "John" Haab, not Johannes. The form also states that she was married thirty years and was a parent of eleven children, "10 are living." At some point in her life she'd felt the sorrow of losing a child.

Her death took place on October 8, 1901, at 7:00 a.m. A local doctor, Theophil Klingmann, looked in on her at home during the last five days of her life. The name listed under "Informant" is Pauline Gross. *The personal and family particulars herein given relative to the deceased are true to the best of my knowledge and belief.* It's the first time I've encountered the human gesture of Pauline's signature. Careful and cramped, it seems to me to be dark with the weight of duty and grief.

In the decade after Kathrina's death, her children not only carry on, but heartily embrace life. Some marry, some have children, some take on new professions, but they always stay close, often working together and caring for each other in order to get by.

Her eldest son, Samuel, marries in 1905. He, his wife and his younger brother Elmer live at the family farm with their father. Samuel takes over as head of household in 1911 after his father dies of chronic bronchitis at the age of seventy.

Emmanuel also marries. He goes from being a clerk in a local department store to co-owning Gross and Dietzel, a shoe shop in Ann Arbor. Pauline and their younger brother Harry live with Emmanuel and his wife Emma during this time. Pauline is listed in the Ann Arbor city directory as a dressmaker, and Harry, a bookkeeper.

My great-grandmother, Tillie, settles in nearby Saline, where her husband, O.C., opens Wheeler's Pharmacy, specializing in drugs, medicines and school supplies. The townsfolk call him "Doc." The newlyweds quickly become pillars of the community. O.C. coaches the local baseball team, is elected town clerk, and belongs to the Masons. Tillie sings in the church choir, belongs to the garden club and the Order of the Eastern Star. In short order they have seven children, five girls and two boys: Katherine (after Kathrina), Grace, Doris, Alice (my grandmother), Elsbeth, Charles and Oscar Jr., who everyone affectionately calls "Bud." Two of Tillie's younger brothers live with them for a time—Walter, while he gets a hardware store up and running; Rudolph, while he finishes school. Their other brother, Albert, works on a farm on the outskirts of town.

In the spring of 1910, Lydia, the eldest sister, suffers a tragic loss. Her husband of twenty years commits suicide, leaving her with nine children to raise, the youngest only three years old. The terrible event is reported on in the *Saline Observer*, Tillie's local newspaper.

A SAD DEATH

Mrs. OC Wheeler last Wednesday received the sad news of the death of her brother-in-law Jacob Stierle of Lima, who ended his life by hanging himself.

Mr. Stierle has had nervous trouble for a long time and although he took treatments at the University hospital, he kept gradually getting worse till at times he had spells when he was not himself. It was Tuesday that one of these spells took him and he committed the terrible deed.

His wife found him in the barn. She had closely watched him since the doctor had told her six months before that Mr. Stierle would suddenly go insane.

He was a faithful Christian and a great church worker.
He had no cause whatever to drive him to commit the deed. The funeral was held Friday, Mr and Mrs OC Wheeler and Walter and Fred Gross attending.   —May 5, 1910

I wonder why the newspaper in the town where Tillie lived ran such a detailed account of her brother-in-law's death. Jacob and Lydia lived a good twenty miles away, and Lydia's name isn't mentioned in the article. Maybe news had travelled quickly from town to town— part lie, part truth—and the writer, sparing sentimentality, was out to set the record straight. Had Tillie orchestrated it from her growing place of influence in the community? Everything my mother ever told me about my great-grandmother points in that direction. Matilda Gross Wheeler was a woman who never shied away from the truth. She preferred to have things out in the open where there was no place for dishonesty to hide. This, to me, is what courage looks like. My mother, who insisted there wasn't room in her life for lies, clearly took after her.

Sin has many tools, but a lie has a handle to fit them all.

I didn't choose to be born with a genetic mutation any more than I chose to have curly hair or hazel eyes, or the likelihood of having lots of freckles, or the predilection for salty over sweet. But I sure as hell can decide which character traits from my ancestors I wish to embrace. Courage, fearlessness, persistence, kindness, a dedication to telling the truth—these are the things I choose.

14.

Junior Mess

Lebanon, Indiana, 1985

"Poise, personality and promise, with an emphasis on excellence. These are the virtues the judges are looking for in this year's Greater Boone County Junior Miss." The pageant organizer is standing behind a lectern at a local community centre, explaining what she expects of her contestants.

I'm in a seat near the back, wondering how I got here. *Maybe I should go.* The chair I'm sitting in is missing the rubber tip off one of its legs and when I move, it makes an angry squawk. Metal versus linoleum, worse than fingernails on a chalkboard. All eyes turn towards me. *One thousand one, one thousand two.* I smile, stay put.

The organizer resumes her speech.

"The categories on which you'll be adjudicated are as follows:
Judges Interview, 35 percent
Creative and Performing Arts, 20 percent
Scholastic Achievement, 15 percent
Poise and Appearance 15 percent
Youth Fitness, 15 percent."

There are any number of similar titles the teenage girls of Indiana can vie for—Pork Queen, Popcorn Festival Queen, Strassenfest Queen, 4-H Fair Queen, Indy 500 Princess. The majority of past winners fit a specific profile: big teeth, blonde hair, long legs, blue eyes, and the ability to act shocked and tearful while having a sash draped over your shoulder and a tiara placed on your head. These are qualities

I don't possess. I'm a short, hazel-eyed brunette who has to bleach her upper lip.

I am Contestant #12.

During a break, Contestant #5 whispers in my ear, "Want to go see *Rocky Horror* tonight? I'll bring the hot dogs and water pistols, you bring the confetti and rice."

She goes to a rival high school, so she doesn't know that I'm a girl with a reputation—for having a crazy grandmother and no steady friends. Though I've known a couple of the contestants since grade school, they treat me as if I'm a complete stranger. As for the rest, some are nice, some are snobbish, some are nightmares in stretch pants and their boyfriends' letter jackets. Contestant #5 seems fun and maybe a little weird like me. "You're on," I tell her. *I guess this won't be so bad after all.*

Who am I kidding? I'm not there for fun. I'm in it for the cash.

I'd already auditioned for music school and been awarded tuition, but I still need to pay for room and books. If I don't raise the money, I'll be going nowhere. My parents can't afford to go into debt for my schooling. Dad's been in the same job for the past twenty years, a sales engineer at a filtration company. The work is steady, the benefits good and his salary fair, but I'd been a surprise baby who'd come along in my parents' late thirties. While their friends are starting to talk of retirement, my folks are still searching for ways to make Dad's paycheque stretch as far as possible.

On top of all that, they have Alice to contend with. In the fallout after the Borax incident, she'd gone to live in a nearby nursing home, where she'd receive proper care when needed, but still have a bit of freedom as well. It had seemed the best solution at the time, but Medicaid doesn't cover all her bills, so my parents have to make up the rest, including the long-distance charges Alice racks up whenever she calls my aunt to complain about her roommate and the staff.

Over the summer Mom and I had both taken part-time jobs at a local flower shop so she could help with bills and I could save for college. Mom works in design and arrangement. I'm a delivery girl. When I'm not schlepping baskets of glads and roses to weddings and

funerals, I'm entering essay contests and pestering my guidance counsellor for scholarship applications. That's how I'd found out about
Junior Miss.

"I don't know if it's right for you," Mom had said, crushing out a
cigarette in an old ceramic ashtray while shaking her head.

Even though her and Dad's roles at home are mostly divided
along traditional gender lines (she cooks the meals, does the laundry
and the shopping; he mows the lawn, fixes the plumbing, changes the
oil in the car), she's a big fan of Gloria Steinem and women's rights.
She's ERA all the way. My sister and I hadn't even been allowed to
play with Barbies. To her, beauty pageants are glorified meat markets.

"It's a scholarship pageant," I explained. "The winner gets money
for the school of her choice."

"Will you have to wear a swimsuit?"

"The competition is based on interview, academics, poise and
appearance, fitness and talent. No swimsuits." (I neglected to tell her
that the fitness portion of the competition consisted of a group dance
number where we'd be required to wear fishnet stockings and over-
sized men's dress shirts.)

Mom looked at the form and then squinted at me over her glasses.
"All right then. Have fun."

Two weeks into rehearsals I'm still struggling, completely out of my
depth. I'd competed in dozens of music competitions over the years
and performed in musicals and plays. I'd even been an extra for a movie
called *Hoosiers* that'd just started filming scenes in my hometown. But
the pageant is something else altogether. Tonight's rehearsal had begun
with the organizer conducting a makeup workshop entitled: "Finding
Your Season." I could give fuck all if I'm a Winter, Spring, Summer or
Autumn. *Fuck all.*

After running through the dance routine, we sit in a circle on the
dusty auditorium floor.

"Ladies," the organizer says, clipboard in hand. "I'm going to go
around the circle and ask you to declare your talent for the

competition. Once I write it down, there's no changing it." She points to Contestant #1.

"Dance, tap," the girl says, popping her gum.

"And you?"

"Dance, ballet."

"And you?"

"Voice solo."

"You?"

"Dance, jazz."

Most of girls are on their school's dance squads and drill teams.

If my aim is to do something that no one else can do, then the rondo from Mozart's 3rd Horn Concerto is my best bet (I'd already played it for my college audition), but as the organizer comes ever closer to calling on me, a French horn solo suddenly seems the least pageant-worthy of all talents.

I sweat as the reckoning continues.

"Dance, modern."

"Piano."

"Dramatic monologue."

"Dance, ballet."

"Dance."

"Dance."

"Dance."

"Contestant number twelve?" The organizer is staring at me, pencil poised.

"Piano, I guess."

Later that night I talk my decision over with Mom as she puts the last touches on my dress for the evening gown competition. She's pieced it together from a few different patterns—cap sleeves, sweetheart neckline, princess waist. I love its retro vibe. It's one of a kind.

"You say there's another girl playing piano?" she asks, pinning a length of lace ribbon to the edge of a sleeve.

"Yes."

"Is she any good?"

"Actually, yeah." I'd heard her noodling around backstage at rehearsal. She had some serious classical chops.

"Then you'll have to do something unexpected. Something she can't." The glint in Mom's eyes is a little unnerving. "Rabid stage-mom" has never been her style.

"The organizer says once we've picked our talent, we can't change our minds. I have to play piano."

"Hmm," she says, motioning for me to step on a wooden footstool so she can check the dress's hem. When she gets halfway around me on her hands and knees she declares, "I've got it! You'll *sing* while you play."

I'd been accompanying myself on piano for years, singing jazz standards and Broadway show tunes, alone or with Alice, but I'd never done it in front of an audience. "I don't know, Mom."

"You'll be fabulous, like Nina Simone or Carole King."

Kate Bush is the first piano-playing songstress that pops into my brain, but I imagine that singing "Wuthering Heights" will get me run off the stage. "Do you have a particular song in mind?"

"You should sing that song by Melissa Manchester that gives me goosebumps."

"Melissa Manchester?" Maybe asking Mom's advice was a mistake.

She stands up, pulls the scrunchie from my hair and fluffs my curls. "You have a similar look. I can already see it. You'll be perfect." She's made up her mind.

She adores the sultry-voiced songwriter. Besides owning all her albums, she'd given me *The Melissa Manchester Songbook* just before last Christmas. "Your present to me this year can be learning to play them."

"Midnight Blue."

"Don't Cry Out Loud."

"The Theme from Ice Castles."

(Please, God, don't let her pick that one.)

"'Come In from the Rain,'" she says. "That's the one I'm thinking of."

It's got lush chords, a killer hook and it sits in the strongest part of my vocal range. "That just might work," I admit.

"Hang on a sec," Mom says dashing to her bedroom. She comes back a few minutes later with my sister's old prom dress draped over her arm. "You should wear this."

Staring at Lori's gown I have a hard time imagining myself wearing it. It's not that the dress is out of style—the shimmery blue satin sheath has an elegant, timeless cut—but Lori is a good three inches taller than I am, and the gown has high slits up the sides and a deep V-neck. I don't see how it will ever fit. I also know we don't have money for another dress.

Mom holds the gown by the shoulders and measures it against me. "We'll have to alter it of course, but by the time I'm through, it'll fit like a glove." Brush rollers bulging under her nylon scarf, she gives me a wink. "Trust me. You can do this."

A week before the pageant I begin to feel as if everything might fall into place. I'm able to make it through the group dance without tripping, I can sing and play my song from memory, and my sister's dress now looks more couture than hand-me-down. I've also seen *The Rocky Horror Picture Show* a half dozen times. Contestant #5 and I laugh and sing through the "Time Warp" during rehearsal breaks.

In the middle of math class one afternoon, my teacher hands me a note. *Please report to the principal's office at once.*

I'm not alarmed. I figure it's just my guidance counsellor with another scholarship application for me to fill out. She's been working overtime on my situation.

I stick my head in her office, but she directs me to the front desk. "Your dad's here," she says. "You'd better go." I can't tell if she's concerned or overworked. Maybe a little of both.

Dad's standing at the desk, hands in his pockets. "Hey there, kiddo."

"What's going on?"

"We're going to the hospital. I'll explain things on the way."

We leave the building in silence.

"Is it Alice?" I ask as we get to the car.

"No, sweetie," Dad says, stopping to unlock my door. "It's your mom, and she's going to be okay."

He's having a hard time looking at me. I don't know what to say.

"Was she in an accident?" I ask. Sometimes she helped out with deliveries at the flower shop during the day.

We both get in the car. "Sort of," he says. "She had a mishap at work."

"Did she fall?"

"She was carrying a box from the storage room when she felt faint. She had a pain in her chest and couldn't breathe. They rushed her to the hospital right away."

My palms go sweaty. "But you said she's going to be okay?"

"Don't worry," he says, starting the engine. "She's already feeling much better. The doctor did an angioplasty. He pushed a little balloon through her blood vessel to clear out a blockage. No surgery required."

I trust Dad on this. If anyone knows how pumps and valves work, it's him.

"When I left she was resting."

"That's good," I say, trying not to panic.

He touches my arm. "I don't want you to be shocked when you see her. She's got a lot of tubes sticking out of everywhere and she's a little groggy from the drugs. But she'll be glad to have you there."

A nurse guides me to a chair beside Mom's bed.

Her face is pale, her eyes, half-closed.

"Hey, Mom," I whisper, worried she's trying to sleep. Dad had tried his best to prepare me, but seeing her like this is terrifying.

She opens her eyes and gives me smile. "Hey there, sweet pea."

I'm nervous and scared and a little weepy. I can't imagine a life without her. "Love you," I say, touching her hand. I think of the words I'd carried in my heart as a child, *Mom is beautiful. Mom is strong. Mom doesn't get sick.*

"They're going to keep me here for a couple of days and then I'll be home. Your dad's going to need your help—cooking dinner, ironing his shirts for work."

I wish Lori were here to help guide me through this, but she's got two kids under five and lives several states away. Her husband works in construction so they've moved four times in as many years: Kentucky, Oklahoma, Georgia, Florida.

"Don't worry about that, Mom," I say. "I'll take care of it."

The nurse checks the bags on the IV drip and leaves.

Mom gives me a reassuring smile. "I'll be home in time to get you ready for the pageant."

"No, Mom," I say. "Let's just concentrate on you getting better. I'll drop out of Junior Miss."

She squeezes my hand tight. "I'm not quitting and neither are you. Giving up isn't something we do."

The evening of the pageant, the dressing room backstage is crawling with mothers armed with bobby pins and mascara. I don't care about any of it. I just want to get through the night.

At intermission I peek from behind the curtains at the side of the stage. I wave to my dad and my brothers, who've come from out of town. Mom's not here. Her doctor wouldn't allow it. She's resting at home, waiting for me.

Changing into my dress for the talent competition, I find a note pinned to the sleeve. *Give 'em goosebumps! Love, Mom.* My name's being called, there's no time for second thoughts or tears. "Contestant number twelve, please take your place." I walk across the stage, sit on the piano bench, put my hands on the keys. I let the spotlight blind my fear. *You are strong. You are brave. You can do this.* By the grace of Melissa Manchester I make it through the song without a single mistake. The audience applauds. One of my brothers hoots, "Way to go, Sis!" I take a brief bow and run off stage.

I have no idea how I get through the evening gown or interview portions of the night, but by the time the whole thing's done, I've won the talent competition and a scholarship for first runner-up.

Contestant #5 catches my arm backstage. "Are you going to the after party?"

"I can't. I need to get home and see my mom."

❋

Tiptoeing into her bedroom, I hold my trophies behind my back.

"Well?" she says. "Don't keep me in suspense."

I place the golden figurines on her bedside table—a young woman with a crown on her head, a treble clef on a music staff. "I didn't take first prize, but I got these."

"Not too shabby," she says with a laugh. "I'm proud of you, sweet pea."

The trophies are nice, but nothing beats hearing her laugh.

"I couldn't have done it without you, Mom."

Mom is beautiful. Mom is strong. Mom doesn't give up.

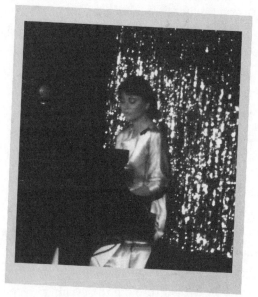

Junior Miss talent competition, 1985

15.

All the Flowers of All Our Tomorrows

Ann Arbor, Michigan, 1913–1919

Love and opportunity serve as guiding stars for Kathrina's children, but there's no escape from the disease that continues to stalk the clan. Eight more members of the extended family die from cancer in less than a decade. Four of them are mothers with young children. One is a young man of twenty-five. His mother dies from the same disease three years later.

Through it all, Pauline continues to refer her relatives to the doctors at the university and relay information to Dr. Warthin. His brash ways haven't quashed her hopes that one day he might find answers for her family.

And now the keen pathologist, who has become head of his department, has announced that a paper he's written about their plight has been accepted for publication. "The world is about to meet Family G," he tells her with a fair bit of pride. "The leading scientific minds of our time are about to have their eyes on you."

"Isn't that something," Pauline says, folding her hands in her lap. *Hopefully one of them will make sense of the things you can't.*

Warthin's "Heredity with Reference to Carcinoma," is published in the *Archives of Internal Medicine* in 1913. In its pages he concludes: "A marked susceptibility to carcinoma exists in the case of certain family generations and family groups." It's the first time Family G is discussed in medical literature but it won't be the last.

Some of the points Warthin makes in the paper are boldly

innovative and he knows it. Confident of his findings, he includes a fair bit of finger-wagging at the medical establishment when it comes to the analysis of cancer, attempting to shame them for not favouring "more trustworthy" histological evidence, like the tissue samples he's been collecting, over clinical diagnoses based merely on signs and symptoms. He also advocates for physicians and surgeons to collect the family histories of cancer patients, insisting that "it is highly desirable that investigations of large family records should be made relative to the occurrence of carcinoma susceptibility."

The latter is the crown jewel of his research. He's used Pauline's pedigree to make a case for his theory of "inherited susceptibility" to cancer. His thinking is that there are families (he cites his own as an example) who are cancer resistant, while others, like Pauline's, who are inordinately susceptible to the disease. To that end, he cites Family G as an example of "a progressive degenerative inheritance—the running-out of a family line through the gradual development of an inferior stock, particularly as far as a resistance to cancer is concerned."

His use of such biting language is no accident. He means to be provocative, and above all, right. Not unlike the renowned founder of eugenics, Sir Francis Galton, who in 1904 wrote in the Journal of American Sociology: "All creatures would agree that it was better to be healthy than sick, vigorous than weak, well-fitted than ill-fitted for their part in life; in short, that it was better to be good rather than bad specimens of their kind, whatever that kind might be. So with men."

Galton's ideas on eugenics have recently found their way into the American consciousness. The belief that supposedly undesirable traits can, and should, be eliminated from the human species by selective breeding is of great interest to social reformers, politicians, scientists and physicians, including Aldred Warthin.

Foundations and societies devoted to the promotion of eugenic principles are springing up across the country. The American Breeders Association sets out to "investigate and report of heredity in the human race and emphasize the value of superior blood and the menace to society of inferior blood." The Eugenics Record Office (ERO) makes it a mission to collect family pedigrees as fuel for lobbying for various solutions to "the problem of the unfit." Scientific Baby and Fitter Family contests pop up at county and state fairs in an effort to normalize the principles of the movement. (Contestants are judged via forms distributed by the ERO; eugenically fit families are awarded "Grade A" status.) Eugenics propaganda posters tout the message: *Some people are born to be a burden to the rest.* A report put forth by the Carnegie Institute explores eighteen methods for removing defective genetic attributes. Method #8 is euthanasia.

Michigan becomes the first state to introduce a compulsory sterilization bill to curtail the procreation of the "unfit." One of the state's most prominent citizens, J.H. Kellogg founds the Race Betterment Foundation in Battle Creek. It's not long before he enlists Warthin in his crusade.

Eager to embrace anything that might lead to thwarting untimely death and disease, the pathologist delivers public lectures on tuberculosis, syphilis, heredity and sanitary reform. He flanks the stalwart knight on his office wall with a pair of woodcuts by Alfred Rethel— *Der Tod als Erwüger* (Death the Strangler) and *Der Tod als Freund* (Death the Friend).

He stares at them frequently, pondering the artist's intentions and marvelling at his skill. The macabre sentinels act as silent companions in the days following his article's publication. His expectations are high as he waits for his peers to respond. He rearranges his desk. He paces the floor. He longs to be lauded more than he cares to admit. *Surely,* he thinks, *they'll see the sense in it all. They'll see that I am right.*

FIRST OF FAMILY TO PASS AWAY

The first break in a family chain of ten members came on Sunday, January 14, 1917, in the death of Elmer A. Gross, who died in an Ann Arbor hospital. He was 28 years old and had lived in Freedom all his life, following the carpenter trade and doing farming.

—*Saline Observer*, January 18, 1917

Cancer came upon Pauline's little brother so suddenly, the doctors had mistaken his symptoms for appendicitis. When the surgeons opened him up to perform an appendectomy, they found his intestines were riddled with cancer. There was nothing they could do to save him.

Dr. Warthin had insisted on performing the autopsy himself.

The following spring, two more young men in the family (one a cousin, the other, Pauline's sister Lydia's eldest son) go the same way as Elmer. They enter the university hospital within twenty-four hours of each other and die two weeks later, on the same day.

In early summer 1919, Pauline takes the pedigree Warthin had included in his paper and begins to amend it. There are mistakes in the chart that she can't abide—wrong dates, missing descendants, incorrect birth orders. He's assured her that none of the errors will nullify his study, but the fastidious dressmaker isn't satisfied until she sets things straight. In the six years since the article was published, there have been several more weddings, births and deaths in the family. She wants the record to be as complete as possible—not a soul forgotten. She feels she herself is running out of time.

It's mid-June, the height of wedding season, her busiest yet. The young men who'd returned from the war the previous autumn had proposed to their sweethearts en masse. Final fittings fill her days, last-minute alterations fill her nights. *Always the dressmaker, never the bride.* She sits at her desk when the day's work is done and continues to add branches and leaves to her family tree. She writes it out in pencil before she commits to pen and ink, applying the same care she takes when making a dress. *Measure twice, cut once.*

Whenever she's got time to spare, she takes the train to visit her sister Tillie and the children in Saline. The four eldest (Katherine, Doris, Alice, Grace) are in their teens now, a quartet of smart, competitive young women who are never at a loss for words. Their three younger siblings, Charlie, Elsbeth and Bud, are full of good-hearted mischief and boundless energy. It's a home filled with laughter and love.

"You're freezing," Tillie tells Pauline as they walk hand in hand in her garden.

"Cold hands, warm heart," Pauline replies.

"And you look a bit pale. Are you unwell?"

"Nothing a good helping of liver and onions won't cure."

"You sound like Mama."

"Good."

Tillie isn't about to let her sister off the hook. "O.C. sells iron pills at the store—'Dr. William's pink pills for pale people.' I'll send Bud down to fetch some for you."

Pauline shakes her head. "Don't trouble the boy with it. He should be off climbing trees or fishing in the river, not waiting on me."

"Are you *sure* you're feeling all right?"

Pauline is far from well. Dark circles have appeared under her eyes and she is tired every morning, even after a good night's sleep. Blessedly, there hasn't been any pain, so she keeps going. She wants to send her last brides off in style, see Tillie's daughter Katherine graduate high school, feel the warmth of the summer sun on her face. "Stop fussing over me. I'm fine."

"I'll call O.C. and ask him to bring the pills home when he closes up for the day. Would you like him to stop by the butcher and get some liver as well?"

Pauline doesn't have the heart to tell her sister what she fears is happening to her. "Thank you, but no, I'm good with just the pills."

On a warm summer day in July, Pauline delivers the finished account of her family's history to Dr. Warthin. Presenting him with the tidy stack of papers, she says, "A present, for you."

Leafing through the pages, he admires her penmanship and her dedication to the cause. "Thank you, Miss Gross. Your help is immeasurable." But he frowns as he counts the number of her kin who have gotten married and had children.

"Something wrong?" Pauline asks. "I've checked every entry several times over."

Warthin shakes his head. "Your work is perfect."

Pauline sits and waits. After twenty-four years, she can tell when there's something weighing on his mind.

Laying the papers aside, he says, "I feel I must repeat what I've made plain to you in the past. Those born into families with a susceptibility to cancer should think long and hard before getting married and having children."

Though his tone is matter-of-fact, she can't help but feel he's looking down his nose at her kin. She won't have it. Their contributions have been great. Their lives have value. "Much can be accomplished, even when life is short," she replies.

"But if suffering can be avoided," he counters. "For the sake of the race."

She glances at the engraving of the knight on the wall. *What does he really stand for? Who is he trying to save?* Pauline's vision of the future isn't a world without her family, it's a world where medical men and scientific minds save them. She understands Warthin well enough to know she won't change his mind. All she can do is hope that someone else will come along and lead the charge. "Good day, Dr. Warthin. Thank you for your time."

"And thank you again for this," he says, laying his hand on the papers. "I'll take good care of it."

Pauline gives a polite nod. *And my family will go on taking care of each other.*

Within days of their meeting, Pauline has to be rushed to the hospital. A biopsy of her womb shows advanced cancer of the uterus. Warthin is in charge of the tissue examination. He's shocked by the rapid onset of the disease. A hysterectomy is ordered at once.

Pauline consents to the surgery, but knows there's little hope. Her worst fears are confirmed when the surgeon discovers cancer has spread from her uterus to parts of her bladder as well. He removes and repairs what he can, then sews her up, leaving a menacing line of stiches across her belly.

In the recovery ward, Tillie sits by Pauline's side. Day after day they talk of their childhood on the farm, and the wonderful time they'd had during their most recent Christmas, when Tillie had gathered much of their family together at her home. Pauline had guessed then that it might be her last.

Tillie brings an armful of fresh flowers from her garden with every visit. Today, it's an enormous bouquet of black-eyed Susans.

A nurse stops her in the hallway before she can enter the room. "Your sister has taken a turn for the worse. She's falling in and out of consciousness. I don't want you to be surprised by her condition."

"How long does she have?" Tillie asks, clutching the flowers to her chest.

"Maybe until day's end. Certainly not much longer."

"Thank you." Tillie moves past the nurse towards her sister.

Pauline gives her a smile as soon as she walks in the room. "Is it my birthday?" she asks, pointing to the flowers.

Tillie can't tell if she's teasing or she's simply lost track of time. It doesn't matter. "Don't I always bring you black-eyed Susies on your special day?" She used to gather them from the pasture for Pauline when they were young. Then they'd sit with their backs against the side of the barn and weave flower crowns.

Pauline whispers, "They're my favourite."

Her birthday isn't for another month. Number forty-seven. Her days are filled with pain. She has a great thirst but no hunger. Her belly feels as if it's on fire. The doctor says that *peritonitis*, caused by a bacterial infection, has settled in her abdomen and is poisoning her blood.

Placing the flowers on a small table, Tillie sits next to the bed. "You should rest," she says. "I'm here."

Pauline nods. "I know."

Tears in her eyes, Tillie bends close and whispers in her ear. "What will I do without you?"

Squeezing her sister's hand, Pauline says, "You'll live."

I've never seen a photograph of Pauline. The only image I have of my great-great-aunt is a magnification of a slide Aldred Warthin made from her tissue samples. If I didn't know what it was, I might mistake it for the marbled endpaper of an antiquarian volume of Charles Dickens or Edith Wharton—*Great Expectations, The House of Mirth*.

No obituary exists for her either. It must've been a last request, to let her go without a fuss, and to be buried in Forest Hill.

But two weeks after her death the following notice appeared in the *Saline Observer*:

MRS. WARTHIN AND MRS. ALFRED LLOYD WERE GUESTS AT THE HOME OF MRS. O.C. WHEELER ON FRIDAY.

Dr. Warthin wasn't with his wife when she and Margaret Crocker Lloyd called on my great-grandmother. Perhaps he thought that delivering condolences was best left to women. Perhaps he feared what Tillie might have to say to him. Perhaps he felt the best way to honour Pauline was through the language he knew best, the language of science.

In a 1925 report titled "The Further Study of a Cancer Family," he writes:

> The writer had also an unusual opportunity of obtaining accurate information concerning various lines of descent in this family from an intelligent and cooperative member of the family, who, unfortunately fell victim herself to a rapidly-developing carcinoma of the uterus. Just before her disease was discovered she had furnished the writer with a complete genealogical table of the family, comprising all of the descendants of the original grand-paternal settler. The present chart, including all descendants, comprises 144 descendants of the original settler.

16.

Homesick

British Columbia and Nova Scotia, November 2017
The pain is sudden, sharp and violent. It takes my breath away. Hand to my belly, I open my eyes to a dark room and stare at the digital display of the alarm clock on the table next to the bed. *12:04 a.m.* The T-shirt I'm wearing is damp with sweat. My forehead's blazing hot, but I'm shaking with chills.

Slowly sitting up, I fight the urge to pass out. The pain I'm feeling isn't accompanied by waves of nausea or gas. It's precise, isolated, intense. I can put my finger on it, three inches up and to the right of my navel. *Fuck.* It won't go away.

I'm alone in a hotel room in downtown Vancouver, six thousand kilometres from home.

Until now the trip had been lovely—a quick mid-November jaunt for book signings, public readings and a few media appearances. At one bookstore, a sweet little girl, maybe five years old, had approached me and tugged on my sleeve. "My mama said I should tell you my name."

I could see her mother, ten feet away, beaming at her daughter.

"She did, did she?"

The girl gave a serious nod.

"All right then, tell me."

"It's Wrennie," she said, before bursting into giggles and running back to her mother.

I motioned for them to come to the table where I'd been signing books. Smiling at the girl, I said, "That's a special name you've got."

"Mama says it comes from one of your books."

"Yes, it does. I gave the name Wrennie to one of my characters because *my* mama used to feed a little wren that built its nest over her bedroom window. The bird went away each winter, but came back every spring. That's because wrens are very smart. They never forget a kindness."

Seeing the two of them together—daughter clutching her mother's hand, mother willing to let her daughter go—had made my heart sing.

I'm not sure if the pain is waning or if I'm just getting used to it, but I decide to get a drink of water and take some Tylenol. If I can manage that, then I'll pace the pain away.

I could call Ian, but it's four in the morning in Nova Scotia. Hearing the phone ring at that hour is its own special hell. I'm not sure how much sense I'd make anyway with this pain gnawing at my brain. Why does Canada have to be so fucking big?

Grabbing my phone I decide to do the thing I know I shouldn't. *This is stupid. This is wrong. Don't do it.* I type my symptoms into Google and search for a diagnosis.

I don't feel like I have to puke or rush to the toilet, so it's clearly not food poisoning or Norwalk virus.

I lift my T-shirt and roughly eyeball the exact location of my pain.

Appendicitis? No.

Gallbladder attack? No.

Biliary colic? No.

Colon cancer? Always a possibility. My mom's doctor had misdiagnosed her onset as the flu.

Don't panic.

I paw through my purse and find a packet of mint tea then boil a pot of water in the room's coffee maker.

I don't want to be like my grandmother, always jumping to the worst conclusion, giving in to fear, wrapping my identity around sickness.

Even if it is cancer, it won't kill me this instant. *Will it?*

I always thought that I'd *know* when it happened, that there would be no doubt in my mind. As the keeper of my family's history,

I figured that I'd gained some sort of spider-sense when it came to identifying cancer in my body. Instead I just feel helpless and confused. I want to go home.

By the time I reach Halifax the next day it's nearly midnight. Ian picks me up at the airport and I collapse into his arms.

The next three days are spent resting and trying to get my body back on track. The pain comes and goes along with fever, chills and night sweats. For a time I stick to stomach-flu protocol, eating only rice, applesauce and bananas before graduating to lacto-fermented pickles, probiotic yogurt and dandelion tea.

Ian had wanted me to go straight to the doctor, but I'd said I wanted to wait a couple of days. From birth to my early thirties I'd been conditioned by the American health care system to avoid doctors whenever possible. Even with insurance they could take a ravenous bite out of your pocketbook if you weren't careful. The first time I'd finished a visit with a doctor in Nova Scotia, I'd gone to the receptionist and opened my wallet. "What do I owe you?" I'd asked, ready to give her my credit card.

She'd given me a blank stare. "Nothing."

"Isn't there anything I have to do?"

Smiling she'd answered, "Have a nice day."

I'd gone to my car, sat in the parking lot and cried.

"You should go see the doctor," Ian chides.

"But I'm starting to feel better," I argue. "It was probably just the flu."

"It's your choice, but I think you'd feel better if you talked some things over with her."

"All right."

"Good. You have an appointment tomorrow, at two."

My doctor chalks it up to a gastrointestinal bug.

I can handle that.

We spend the rest of the appointment catching up on my yearly previvor to-do list.

"I've put in a request for a colonoscopy with a new gastroenterologist. I'm not sure how long the wait will be, though."

"I'm not due for a while yet. I had one this past January."

She types some notes on her laptop, prints out an order for blood work. "Just the usual tests. I need to see if anything's out of whack."

We schedule a dermatology exam, chat about mammograms, put an order in for a transvaginal ultrasound so we can check on my ovaries. (My to-do list was even longer when I still had a uterus.)

"Hop up here so I can take your blood pressure," she says once we've gotten through the list.

I sit on the examination table and roll up my sleeve.

I try to stay calm and breathe deep as the cuff slowly squeezes my arm.

The doctor shakes her head. "It's a little high today."

I shrug and say, "White coat syndrome?"

"Possibly."

"It's nothing personal."

She laughs.

Putting the buds of her stethoscope in her ears, she listens to my heart. "Hmm," she says then moves the end of the stethoscope to the side of my neck and listens again. She moves it to the other side and does the same.

"What is it?" I ask.

"I'm pretty sure you have a heart murmur."

"What?" That's definitely not something I thought I'd hear today.

Sitting at her desk she starts typing again. "We'll need to order more tests . . . to see what's causing it."

"Sure," I say. "Anything I need to know in the meantime?"

"If you have chest pains or are short of breath for no reason, get to the hospital at once. Barring that, try not to worry. It could be totally innocent. We'll get to the bottom of it."

What if I can't bear one more thing?

17.

Graduation

Terre Haute, Indiana, 1991

I'm twenty-two and completely intoxicated by all that comes with late spring in a Midwestern college town. Long walks in the sycamores along the river. Late-night conversations on crumbling, tumble-down porches. Fevered dancing to music that pulses through my veins— REM, Depeche Mode, XTC, Tori Amos. I want to be like Tori— electric, shameless, fearlessly sexual, an angry girl writhing behind a piano refusing to sit still.

Hair pulled in a messy topknot, wrinkled T-shirt smelling of stale patchouli and incense, I stumble out of bed, parched and wilted from the previous night's revels. The stress of exams is over and graduation is on the horizon. I've made it through the maze of term papers, study groups, dress rehearsals, faculty juries, and end-of-semester performances that make up my life as a music major. I've got plenty of cause for celebration.

Standing at the window, I watch a flurry of magnolia petals fall from the sprawling tree outside my apartment. Bruised, helpless beauties caught in the wind on the wrong side of town. My boyfriend stirs and groans in my bed, pulls a sheet over his face, hiding from the morning sun. I have a terrible habit of falling in love at the end of the term.

We'd sat next to each other in orchestra all semester, shuffling scores, sharing pencils, conspiring over breath marks. I was determined not to give in to his Ferris-Buelleresque charms, but when the conductor put Brahms' third symphony in front of us, everything went sideways. French horn players become masterful flirts when they've got nothing to do but count rests for measures on end. Now he wants me to move in with him.

I don't know what I want, at least not when it comes to love. My focus has been on my schoolwork and deciding what comes next. I've just been awarded a TA position in the music department along with a scholarship towards a graduate degree in musicology. If that works out, maybe I'll get a PhD.

I love my life at the university. Mom had been right, I did find my tribe—clowns, divas, music geeks, kindred spirits, a family of my choosing. I've become confident and happy. By day, I'm steeped in the world of Brahms, Beethoven, Schoenberg and Stravinsky. By night, I sneak off to hole-in-the-wall dives for open mics and jazz.

"Hey, sleepyhead," I say, sitting on the edge of the bed, nudging the Boyfriend awake. "You in there?"

"Mmmhmm." He grabs my arm, tries to pull me into bed.

I look at the clock. It's edging on ten. "You can stay as long as you like, but I've got to go."

Running a brush through my hair, I pin it up, then slip into my latest Salvation Army find. It's a stunner of a vintage dress, shirred lavender chiffon with a halter neck, reminiscent of Elizabeth Taylor circa 1951. Reminiscent of my mom, who was a freshman at Michigan State that same year. I wonder how I'd look with a beauty mark and short hair. *Shit, it's 10:30.* The Honors Day convocation starts in less than an hour. I'm getting a medal for the grad scholarship and my honor cords for graduating cum laude. Good thing I'm not meeting up with my parents until after it's over. Good thing the Boyfriend isn't coming along. Mom can always tell what the outcome of my relationships will be the minute she meets whatever guy I'm dating. If she thinks the Boyfriend is a loser, I'll see it in her face. I swear she's able to mark the date of my breakups on her calendar months in advance. This boyfriend is shiny and new, still in test-drive mode. I'll hold off on subjecting him to Mom's eagle eye for a little longer.

❧

The convocation is stuffy, hot and boring, and I'm glad when it's over. I wave to some friends who'd gotten roped into playing in a string quartet for the reception, then make my way through the crowd to find my folks.

They've been incredibly supportive throughout my college years, regularly making the long trek from home to attend concerts, recitals and performances. Mom has been especially invested in it all. This milestone means as much to her as it does to me. She'd never had that kind of support from Alice when she was in school. I've seen the letters to prove it. Every page Alice sent to my mom while she was away is laced with passive-aggressive bids for pity or praise. She never asks about her daughter's well-being or whether there is anything she needs. Instead, she barrages her with constant reminders of their fractured bond.

> I've been trying to figure out how we can get along better.
> I know I'm at fault in a lot of ways, but don't seem to know how to go about helping it.

These days Alice was at arm's length, only visiting the house during holidays and family get-togethers. She'd learned to be comfortable at the nursing home, and thankfully that had led to her being less bent on yanking Mom's chain.

Spying my parents near the exit, I head in their direction. When I reach them, Dad gives me a hug. "I'm proud of you, kiddo."

Mom chimes in, "We both are."

"Thanks," I say. Flashing the medal hanging around my neck, I ask, "How about we go get some lunch? It's on me."

Dad looks to Mom. "Can we take a rain check? We'd like to get home before supper."

As we walk out of the building and into the noonday sun, I can see how pale Mom is. She's holding tight to Dad's arm, more for support than out of affection. "Are you feeling okay?" I ask.

Taking a seat on a bench on the sidewalk, she motions for me to sit next to her. "I had a long day yesterday."

"We were at the hospital," Dad says.

I put my arm around her shoulder. "Why didn't you tell me you weren't feeling well? You didn't have to come today." I'm trying not to jump to any conclusions.

"I didn't want you to worry. You've had so much on your plate. There was no sense in saying anything until we had all the facts."

Dad steps in again. He's angry, but not with Mom. "We would've known what was wrong a lot sooner if it hadn't been for that quack of a doctor."

"Larry," Mom scolds. "Calm down."

"I won't," he says, turning red in the face. "That goddamned doc refused to take your mother's family medical history seriously. He thought he knew better. First he said it was the flu, then he said it was an ulcer, then he said maybe it was adhesions from the hysterectomy your mom had when she was thirty-eight. All the while your poor mother was doubled over with pain and unable to eat. This went on for a month! She could put her finger on the spot where it hurt. She begged him for a colonoscopy. She knew all along."

"Anyway," Mom interrupts. "I went to emergency yesterday and got it done."

"A colonoscopy?"

"Yes."

My heart sinks. "Is it cancer?"

Dad cuts to the chase. "The mass in her cecum is so large they couldn't get the scope all the way through. They had to follow up with a barium X-ray. She's going in for surgery day after tomorrow."

Mom tries to lessen the blow. "You'd like the doctor who was on call. She's very good. After I came back from my tests, she gave me a smack on the fanny and said, 'I'll see you in surgery.' Then I asked if she could wait a couple days more so I could at least go to your Honors Day. She wouldn't let me wait any longer than that."

I'm reeling with how insane this all sounds. "God, Mom. I can't believe you're even here right now. How about I come home with you and stay for as long as you need me. I don't have to go to commencement."

"Nonsense," Mom scolds. "You'll do no such thing. Come home for a couple of days if you like, but promise me you'll walk across that stage."

"Maybe. I don't know. Let's just wait and see."

"No. You're going. Promise me."

Dad gives a helpless shrug. "You'd better give her what she wants. She won't take no for an answer."

"All right," I say. "I promise."

When I was sure Mom was in the clear after her surgery, I went back to school to don my cap and gown. Dad and both my brothers came for commencement along with my sisters-in-law and my niece and nephew. My sister stayed with Mom.

The next day I drove home to watch the videotape of the big day with her. When it was over, I helped her get dressed and fix her hair. She'd insisted I bring my cap and gown home so Dad could take our picture together.

"Oh, dear," she said, holding on to the top of her slacks. She'd lost so much weight her pants wouldn't stay up. "Grab a safety pin from my sewing kit and pin the waist."

I fiddle with the waistband until it's snug. "Dad says you'll be getting chemo. Do you know when that will start?"

"Soon," she says. "I don't want to wait around."

"I understand."

Taking a tube of lipstick from her nightstand she takes the lid off, twists the tube and swipes it across her lips. She's not going to let anything stop her. Not today, not ever.

We're both staring into the mirror when she confesses, "After I came home from the hospital, all I wanted was to take a shower. When I got out I looked at myself and I thought 'You're a real mess.' And then your dad came in and sat on the floor and dried my feet. He even got between my toes. That was the moment I decided I wasn't going to let this beat me. I have this man who's willing to take care of me no matter what, and I don't want to let him down.

"I thought all my life that I'd probably have to deal with this. It didn't come as a surprise, but it does make me angry as hell. Cancer had better watch out, because I'm going to kick its ass."

I believe her.

Standing in front of a blue spruce in the front yard, Mom and I squint back the sun and smile for the camera.

Dad says the magic words he's been saying all my life. "Would you look at your mother? Isn't she just the prettiest gal you've ever seen?"

Holding Mom's hand I say, "Yes, she is."

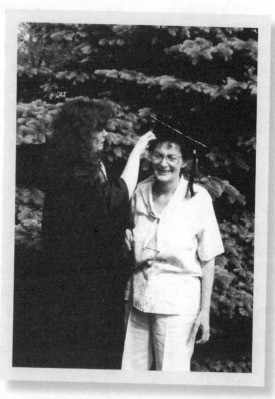

Me and Mom, post-graduation, 1991

18.

Dimples and Cupid Bow Lips

Ann Arbor, Michigan, 1920–1931

After Pauline's death, Warthin uses her revised pedigree as the basis for a second, more complete report. "The Further Study of a Cancer Family" is published in the *Journal of Cancer Research* in 1925.

His initial article hadn't gained him the recognition he'd hoped for, and his rancour is evident in the text of his new one: "When this study was reported it met with little favor among surgical writers and particularly among those interested in propaganda for the prevention of cancer. In some of the literature put out under this latter head, the statement was made that there was no evidence of a familial susceptibility to cancer."

Most surgeons are far more interested in developing new and efficient treatment practices and techniques than they are in Warthin's theory of inherited susceptibility. When it comes to progressive medical thought surrounding cancer, they've aligned themselves with the newly formed American Society for the Control of Cancer (ASCC) and their Do Not Delay campaign. This is the "propaganda" Warthin takes to task in his report.

He can't prove *why* a tendency towards certain cancers occurs in some families, only that his statistics support his hunch that such tendencies exist. Science simply hasn't come up with the tools to confirm his theory yet.

The ASCC wants to steer away from talk of a hereditary predisposition to cancer. Being diagnosed with cancer is considered a death sentence. Fear and shame surrounding the disease is so pervasive that patients often keep their illness a secret from their families. Some doctors even go so far as to withhold test results from their patients. If people are told that they're preordained to get cancer, the ASCC believes, many will become so troubled by the notion, they'll ignore symptoms when they arise, and refuse to seek medical care. Their Do Not Delay campaign is designed to destigmatize the disease while kicking the door open to public discourse about cancer. If they can raise awareness in the general population about the importance of recognizing symptoms and seeking early surgical intervention, then they can save lives.

Warthin takes the ASCC's position as a personal affront. He uses the rhetoric of the eugenics movement to form his own "biological philosophy," which he freely shares with all who will listen.

DIMPLES AND CUPID BOW LIPS, BEAUTY OR LOW INTELLIGENCE?

Is the dimple a mark of beauty? Or is the maid with that bewitching birthmark and Cupid's bow mouth less beautiful and intelligent than her sister without those attractions?

Dr. A.S. Warthin, eminent pathologist of the University of Michigan says they bear a relationship to the harelip and cleft palate, which never yet in this or any other land have been accepted as beautiful. They mark a girl as "below par" says Dr. Warthin.

He said it during a lecture on "The Inheritance of Disease," in which he made a direct appeal for eugenics, better living conditions that should breed better humans, and a plea for the recognition of certain inheritances.

He declares that "blood will tell" has proven its truth throughout the ages and that today this fact was becoming recognized and that civilized people were at least considering what could be done to breed a better race.

"Today it is recognized that all men are not born equal. We are not equal so far as the value of our bodily cells is concerned."

—Ann Arbor, Michigan, September 5, 1922

Accounts of Warthin's lecture appear in newspapers across the United States, from large cities to small towns, coast to coast, including the editions Tillie's husband, O.C., sells in his drugstore.

The well-spoken pathologist becomes a popular attraction on the public-speaking circuit, drawing large crowds and high praise. Local organizations and church groups tout his stereoscopic presentations. His old friend J.H. Kellogg and other leaders within the eugenics movement are thrilled to have him in their camp. As a respected university professor, head of his department, and past president of the American Association of Pathologists, Warthin is an invaluable asset to their cause, joining the cadre of scientists from prestigious universities who are actively introducing "race theory" and "race science" into their classrooms.

The enormous influx of immigrants arriving in America during the past decade has caused a perfect storm where race fears and class bias have combined to create an atmosphere of bigotry and discrimination. Those most active in funding the movement are society's elite—members of the Carnegie Institute, the Rockefeller Foundation, and the Harriman Railroad dynasty—all believing that wealth equals virtue; poverty equals poor character; and illness a sure sign of genetic weakness. They use their influence to sway politicians to enact laws authorizing the sterilization of citizens with "hereditary defects," including epilepsy, criminality and alcoholism. Cancer is among the conditions the movement seeks to define as "hereditary," and, therefore, socially unacceptable. In the coming decades thirty-two states will adopt such laws, and seventy thousand Americans will be sterilized against their will.

Women's groups and charitable organizations such as the Woman's Christian Temperance Union also take up the banner of eugenics under the guise of "social betterment." They encourage their members to study the principles of heredity and social hygiene. Premarital genetic fitness tests that include family histories are highly encouraged. A popular short film of the day is titled: *Are You Fit to Marry?*

It's a question that's been on Warthin's mind since he'd first laid eyes on Pauline's family tree. *No*, he still thinks, *in a perfect world, those*

*with an inherited susceptibility to disease should not marry and have fam-
ilies.* Pauline's death hasn't softened his views in the least. If anything,
it has made him more strident.

Throughout the 1920s, the Rockefeller Foundation donates over a
half-million dollars towards the establishment of a eugenics program in
Germany. Various organizations in the American eugenics movement
supply German officials and scientists with literature concerning their
agenda. In the pages of *Mein Kampf,* Hitler praises the American
approach of using eugenics to shape immigration. "There is today one
state in which at least weak beginnings toward a better conception [of
immigration] are noticeable. Of course, it is not our model German
Republic, but the United States." He also confides to a Nazi comrade,
"I have studied with great interest the laws of several American States
concerning prevention of reproduction by people whose progeny would,
in all probability, be of no value or be injurious to the racial stock."
Germany's sterilization rate will eventually grow to more than five
thousand per month. Joseph DeJarnette, superintendent of Virginia's
Western State Hospital, comments in the *Richmond Times-Dispatch,*
"The Germans are beating us at our own game."

In January of 1927 at a "Race Betterment" conference in Battle
Creek, Michigan, Warthin boldly interrupts the proceedings to proclaim to the several hundred delegates present that the papers they've
been presenting are more suited to a "race deterioration conference" than
a race betterment discussion. Bullying his way to the lectern he declares,
"What the world truly needs is a new religion, a new philosophy of life.
If the race is to improve, the choice of a life mate on the basis of love or
sex attraction alone must stop. Two young people preparing to wed
should make some investigation into the past life of the proposed life
partner and into the lives of his or her ancestors and find out whether or
not there are conditions which may result in disaster to their children."

After the conference is over, Warthin forcefully reiterates his
position in his writing: "The State should require eugenic marriages
and prevent non-eugenic ones. No individual should be allowed to
produce children who possess a germ-plasm so seriously below par as
to make him an undesirable citizen."

These eugenic ideas will remain the guiding principles of Warthin's work for the rest of his life.

In January of 1931, Tillie opens the morning paper to find the following headline: "Cancer Cures Deplored By University Physician."

The *Saline Observer* has published excerpts from an article Warthin had written for *Annals of Internal Medicine*. In it, he bemoans the rise in popularity of cancer cures sold by quack physicians. He also proclaims, yet again, that the first and foremost "line of attack" against cancer is "breeding out the inherited family strains, which requires a wider popular faith in eugenics than prevails."

Someday, Tillie thinks, *we'll prove him wrong.*

Warthin's last written work isn't a scientific paper, but a scholarly monograph titled *The Physician of the Dance of Death*. In it, he catalogues and comments on a personal collection he's amassed over the course of his career—over 685 books, etchings and other works of art depicting Death. "This study of man's changing physical reactions to the concept of Death, throughout six centuries, has occupied the writer, in his scattered hours of leisure, affording him much stimulating interest and mental recreation." Of the one thousand copies that are printed, one hundred are specially bound, to be given by Warthin as gifts to his friends and colleagues. The frontispiece is none other than Albrecht Dürer's *Knight, Death and the Devil*, the sixteenth-century engraving he'd kept by his desk his entire career. *Across my path though Hell should stride, / Through Death and Devil I will ride.*

The German philosopher Friedrich Nietzsche, too, was an admirer of Dürer's knight and gifted a print of the engraving to composer Richard Wagner as a representation of a "brave future." During the rise of the Third Reich, members of the Nazi party would come to idealize Dürer as "the most German of all artists." Dürer's knight was used in their propaganda as the image of a racially pure, Aryan ideal.

Each of the special edition copies of *The Physician of the Dance of Death* is accompanied by Warthin's "biological creed," his personal manifesto professing his devotion to eugenics.

CREDO

I believe in the law.

In the immortality of the germ plasm and in the creative-progressive evolution of life. In the variability of value of the germ plasm through heredity and environment. In the transmission of acquired characters. And in the conscious improvement of the race through the laws of volitive eugenics. I believe that the aim of the individual life is the protection, improvement and continuation of the immortal germ plasm. And that this is best secured by self-development in the highest possible degree through a permanent monogamic sex-partnership with limitation of offspring towards the securing of the best possible results in the progeny, and their best preparation for the continuation of the process in the next generation. In this belief, the universe is rationalized for my intelligence and reason. I accept it with optimism, relinquishing all desire for a personal immortality, and, unafraid, believing that whatever gods may be, the game of life will have been played squarely and according to the law.

In the spring of 1931, Aldred Scott Warthin dies unexpectedly of a sudden asthma attack.

The last Family G case he studies comes a mere month before his passing, when Tillie is diagnosed with advanced uterine cancer. Although Warthin doesn't live to see the long-term results, Tillie's case will be the most remarkable yet.

19.

Lebkuchen and Life

Scots Bay, Nova Scotia, December 2017
Copy number ninety-three of *The Physician of the Dance of Death* sits on the shelf above my writing desk. It's bound in robin's egg blue, with the title and Warthin's name embossed in gold.

If Warthin had gotten his way, I wouldn't be alive.

I let that sink in and wrap its wormy truth around my heart.

I don't want to despise him, but I do. And I hate myself for it. This is not who I am. It's not how I was raised. History would have me think he was a patient man, a man who listened, a man who heard truth in Pauline's words. End of story. Except for the part of the tale that lives on in me, whispering, *You're broken, unfixable, a mistake.*

I'm saddened by the discovery that he promoted such toxic ideas, but more than that, I'm angry.

I'm angry for all those who were made to feel lesser because of him.

I'm angry for my ancestors who heeded his words and chose not to marry. Who looked after their heartbreak, their anguish?

I'm angry because history, once again, has relegated a woman to the footnotes, ignoring her contributions and courage.

I'm angry because the story history has chosen to tell about this man is built on a dangerous amnesia, born of a country that continually chooses to forget its failings, mistakes and sins.

Those who cannot remember the past are doomed to repeat it.

❧

Two weeks before Christmas my eldest son comes home for a visit. His little brother and I have spent the day in the kitchen baking leb-kuchen. Legend says that monks, who lived in the Swabian region of Germany, first made the now-traditional treat during the thirteenth century. My family's recipe has been passed down from my great-great-grandmother Kathrina, to Tillie, to my great-aunt Doris, to my mother, to me. The deliciously dense cookie is laden with honey, molasses, spices, candied fruit and nuts. It was the only food that soothed my stomach when I suffered from morning sickness during both of my pregnancies.

"I think I should test one," Eldest Son says, angling to snitch a cookie from a cooling rack in the kitchen.

His brother gives him a sideways glare. He knows the recipe clearly states, *Don't eat for two weeks, Gram Tillie's law.*

Rather than scrawling the instructions on 3x5 index cards, my mother had meticulously recorded them on three sheets of lined note-paper before giving the recipe to me. She also included several do's and don'ts from the various recipe bearers over the past century.

A pint's a pound the world 'round.

If buttermilk's not to be found, sour fresh with vinegar.

Don't make this on a day you just cleaned the kitchen . . .

"Mom?" Youngest Son asks. He's never been a rule breaker.

I hand a cookie to each of them. "For quality assurance. I'm sure Tillie wouldn't mind." If the cookies make it to Christmas Day, they'll see that she was right. Lebkuchen is best when the spices have had time to settle, mix and mingle.

"Hey," Eldest Son says, handing me an envelope. "I brought you an early Christmas present.

It's from the Maritime Human Genetics Research Centre in Halifax.

"They sent me some forms to fill out so I can get tested. I was going to do it by myself, but I need a little help."

Opening the envelope, I look over the forms. "No problem," I say, grabbing a pen. "Let's get 'er done."

We fill in the family medical history, line by line, cancer by cancer, relative by relative. I write a cover letter to include with the forms that briefly outlines our long history with Lynch syndrome.

Once it's all tucked in an envelope, sealed, addressed and stamped, I turn to him and ask, "You doing okay with this? It's one thing to say you'll get tested, it's quite another to take the leap."

"The woman from the testing centre was great, really easy to talk to, very helpful and informative."

"Good." It's a relief to see him so calm, positive and upbeat. "Did she say how long you'll have to wait until they call you for a blood draw?"

"Up to a year, but hopefully much sooner."

"I'm proud of you, kiddo."

"Thanks, Mom."

That night I can't sleep. I lie in bed and pray that I've given him all he needs to deal with this—intellectually, emotionally, spiritually. My wish, of course, is that the results will be negative, but my mind runs wild imagining what will happen if the results go the other way. What will I do? What will I say? I need to be there for him. I need to do the right thing. I want him to know how much he's loved.

Slipping out of bed I go to my desk to search for another piece of paper that bears my mother's handwriting. It's a letter she wrote after I received my test results—another recipe of sorts, a recipe for life.

May 13, 2002

Darling,

I don't think there ever has been a time in my life when I couldn't come up with the right words before today. My heart was so full of guilt and sadness, then joy and gladness. I didn't think it would happen that way. You know how moms are. They want to take all the bumps for their kids and make every bruise better.

My great joy is that you are a beautiful intelligent woman who loves life and will do everything you can to keep yourself healthy. This is a challenge to hit head on. Visualize yourself dressed in football gear, tackling the thing and winning.

Well enough of this. Let's go forward.

Love you,

Mom

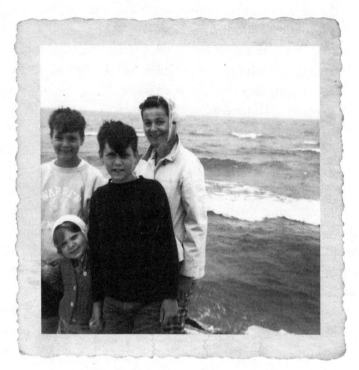

Mom with Skip, Doug and Lori, 1967

To not know
what happened
before you were
born is to remain
forever a child.

—Cicero

II.

Love. Courtship. Birth.

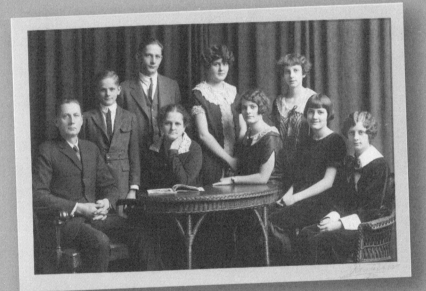

Previous page: Tillie, O.C. and family, 1928

20.

Knowings

Saline, Michigan, 1931
It's late March, two weeks before Easter. As crocuses stage joyful riots of colour in churchyards and front lawns, every tree, shrub and blade of grass strives towards green ecstasy.

All creatures of our God and King; lift up your voice and with us sing.

All this growth, tenderness, vigour and faith stirs the townsfolk to their annual rites of spring—church picnics, fish fries, baseball practices, garden club meetings, over the fence tête-à-têtes.

Oh praise Him! Alleluia!

Tillie stands outside her husband's pharmacy, hair swept back in a tidy bun, hands tucked in her apron pockets, glasses sliding down the bridge of her nose. Above her head a large neon sign creaks on a metal frame. WHEELER'S DRUGS, EST. 1901. She's scrutinizing a spring gardening display she's just installed in the storefront window. *Something's missing,* she thinks as her eyes flit from object to object—a pair of ladies' garden gloves, a copy of the *Farmer's Almanac,* a shiny trowel with a sturdy wooden handle, a straw sunhat artfully laid beside a trio of terracotta flower pots. In front of the last pot, she'd placed a small sign from her favourite seed company, D.M. Ferry and Co.

HOW DOES YOUR GARDEN GROW?

Something's not right.

The morning breeze is warm and steady, carrying the scent of fresh-turned earth from the farmland on the outskirts of town. Eyes closed, Tillie recalls the spring mornings of her childhood when the twitter of swallows mingled with her sister's laughter as she and Pauline chased each other beneath the patchwork quilts and calico skirts their mother had strung on the clothesline to dry. *That's it!* she thinks, plan hatched. *That's what it needs.* Entering the shop, she goes to the counter and pulls a length of twine from the cast-iron holder that sits next to the till, catching the end with her toe and measuring it against herself. Five foot two. (But her eyes aren't blue. They're brown.) After snipping the twine, she searches for hammer and nails in a toolbox her husband keeps under the counter, then grabs a package of clothespins from the shelf and empties it into the left pocket of her apron. Then she steps over to a tall wooden rack and chooses several envelopes of seeds: delphinium, calendula, nasturtium, hollyhock, cabbage, snap pea, carrot, broccoli, lettuce, turnip, beet, cucumber, sunflower, snapdragon and three kinds of beans—lima, wax and pole. If her husband, who is making a morning round of deliveries while she minds the shop, complains about the clothespins or the seed packets, she'll simply remind him of the steep price they paid for the neon monstrosity of a sign. The gaudy, buzzing thing had made the social column of the *Saline Observer* the day after it'd been installed. "A fine new sign," the paper had declared, in bold print no less. The thought of it still rankles her. Times have been tough for most people since the Crash of '29, and it feels like bad form to make any display of success. People's pocketbooks are dry.

"But does it have to be so big?" she'd asked her husband when it first went up.

"It brightens up the street," O.C. had said, grinning, nudging her with his elbow. "We can all use a little cheer right about now, don't you think?"

"I suppose."

Tillie knows that her husband isn't a frivolous man. He was simply trying his best to improve business. And she's fairly certain that no one in all of Washtenaw County has ever said a disparaging word about him, and they probably never will.

A good pharmacist (which he is) has to know as much about medicine as any doctor, and as much about human frailty as any man of the cloth. O.C. has been in the buisness for thirty years. People trust the man they call "dear old Doc." What's more, they like him. By day he fills prescriptions, gives sound advice, lectures kids who steal lemon drops from the candy bin about what it means to have good character. Evenings, after supper, twice a week, April through October, he makes his way to the local baseball diamond to coach a team of rowdy boys. Friday nights, year-round (more often than Tillie would like), he drives an old delivery truck to the shacks and hollows on the edge of town where men congregate to drink moonshine and gamble things they can't afford to lose. Rather than joining them—though he takes an occasional nip—he hauls them safely home, immune to their proclivity for drunkenness and fistfights, half-baked excuses, and wetting themselves while cursing the local fat cats and big wigs. Once he's delivered the last offender to his doorstep, he's home in time to exchange greetings with the milkman. Kissing Tillie on the forehead as he at last climbs into bed, he always whispers, "Good morning, Mrs. Wheeler." After thirty years of marriage, it still makes her blush.

Perching herself on a stepstool, she hammers in a nail on opposite sides of the front window's frame, strings the twine between them, then pins the seed packets to the line. When she's finished, the display is as bright and cheerful as any string of pennants proclaiming Happy Birthday! Welcome Home! Go Team!

There's a practical side to what she's doing as well. The display is meant to entice customers to purchase the simple gardening supplies they carry, and, more importantly, to plant a garden so they can provide for themselves during hard times. *So many have so little. Who knows when it will end.* With a handful of change and fair bit of sweat, a person can grow enough vegetables to stock their pantry shelves for the winter. That was what her mother had done to keep their family fed—preserving, pickling, jamming and relishing everything in sight. Tillie, in turn, has done the same for her brood. It takes effort, but the rewards are great, giving comfort, relief and satisfaction as well as sustenance. The flowers, of course, are for Beauty's sake.

All the flowers of all our tomorrows are in the seeds we plant today.

Coming down off the stepstool she feels a twinge of pain, below her belly, deep inside.

Something's not right.

It burns for an instant as she holds her breath, then subsides. It's happened before. Last time, she found afterward that her best slip was spotted with blood.

It's probably nothing.

Inside, she glances at her reflection in the mirror behind the counter. The grey streaks in her hair seem to have multiplied overnight and the lines across her brow grown deeper. Is that a liver spot on her cheek? She swears it wasn't there when she'd gotten dressed this morning. *Where is the girl who used to be me?* She'll celebrate her fifty-fifth birthday in June, God willing.

Mama died at fifty-five.

There are no women left in her family to commiserate with or to ask for advice. Pauline has been gone over a decade, and Lydia died three years ago this past October. She's the last daughter standing. Her brother Emmanuel is gone now too, leaving his dear wife, Emma, to carry on without him. (They had no children. A blessing, curse, or choice?) Of her parents' ten children, only half survive—Walter, Albert, Rudolph, Samuel and herself. Cancer has cruelly picked off the rest. *Who will be next?*

At least Samuel still has the farm. If they were to lose that too, she doesn't think she could bear it. All her best memories from childhood are rooted in that place, from a time when the world was right and the ground beneath her feet felt solid and sure.

"I need to go to talk to a man about soybeans," Samuel had said as they'd strolled through the main exhibition hall at last summer's State Fair.

"Soybeans?" Tillie had asked. "I thought we were here to relive old memories—to do the things we used to do when we were young."

"Look at farm equipment we can't afford?"

"Eat ice cream. Listen to the codgers argue about the weather."

"Guess I'm a codger now, myself," he'd teased. "I won't be long. I'll meet you outside when I'm done."

While she was waiting, Tillie took a stroll past the many booths that lined the hall, stopping occasionally to look at something that caught her eye—a demonstration of a new type of percolating coffee pot; a display of the latest varieties of sunflowers on offer from D.M. Ferry and Co. with the booth attendants handing out free samples. Seed packets in hand, she'd nearly reached the exit when she spotted a large banner hanging between the Pressman's Union booth and the International Harvester display.

FITTER FAMILIES CONTEST

AND EUGENICS EXHIBIT

SPONSORED BY:

THE AMERICAN EUGENICS SOCIETY

Every inch of the booth was covered with placards.

HOW LONG ARE WE AMERICANS TO BE SO CAREFUL FOR THE PEDIGREE OF OUR PIGS AND CHICKENS AND CATTLE; AND THEN LEAVE THE ANCESTRY OF OUR CHILDREN TO CHANCE, OR "BLIND" SENTIMENT?

"SELECTED" PARENTS WILL HAVE BETTER CHILDREN.

THIS IS THE AIM OF EUGENICS. IF ALL MARRIAGES WERE EUGENIC, WE COULD BREED OUT MOST UNFITNESS IN THREE GENERATIONS.

GOOD HEREDITY: ARE YOU A THOROUGHBRED? SEE HOW YOUR FAMILY COMPARES WITH THE

NATIONAL EUGENIC STANDARDS.
FITTER FAMILIES EXAMINATIONS GIVEN HERE.

Dead centre was a series of signs, each fitted with a flashing light.

THIS LIGHT FLASHES EVERY 15 SECONDS:
EVERY 15 SECONDS $100 OF YOUR MONEY GOES
FOR THE CARE OF PERSONS WITH BAD HEREDITY
SUCH AS THE INSANE, FEEBLEMINDED, CRIMINALS
AND OTHER DEFECTIVES.

THIS LIGHT FLASHES EVERY 48 SECONDS:
EVERY 48 SECONDS A PERSON IS BORN IN THE
UNITED STATES WHO WILL NEVER GROW UP
MENTALLY BEYOND THAT STAGE OF A NORMAL 8
YEAR OLD BOY OR GIRL.

THIS LIGHT FLASHES EVERY 50 SECONDS:
EVERY 50 SECONDS A PERSON IS COMMITTED TO
JAIL IN THE UNITED STATES.
VERY FEW <u>NORMAL</u> PERSONS EVER GO TO JAIL.

THIS LIGHT FLASHES EVERY 16 SECONDS:
EVERY 16 SECONDS A PERSON IS BORN IN THE
UNITED STATES.

THIS LIGHT FLASHES EVERY 7 ½ MINUTES:
EVERY 7 ½ MINUTES A HIGH GRADE PERSON IS
BORN IN THE UNITED STATES WHO WILL HAVE
THE ABILITY TO DO CREATIVE WORK AND BE FIT
FOR LEADERSHIP. ABOUT 4% OF AMERICANS COME
WITHIN THIS CLASS.

SOME PEOPLE ARE BORN TO BE A BURDEN
TO THE REST.

A pretty young woman stood at the side of the booth, waiting to pounce. Honey-blonde hair pinned away from her face, she was smiling and holding a clipboard. Her white dress, simply cut and neatly pressed, gave her the clean, no-nonsense look of a nurse. "Would you like me to assess your health?" she asked. "It's free of charge."

Tillie was too stunned to reply.

Pointing to a silver loving cup on a nearby table, the young woman continued her spiel. "We'll be awarding this fine Governor's trophy to the Fittest Family in the state at the end of the week. Perhaps that family is yours?"

Tillie shook her head. *This can't be real.* "My family isn't with me," she said.

Pulling a shiny bronze medallion from her pocket, the girl pressed on. "Not to worry," she said, handing it to Tillie. "Individuals who demonstrate outstanding constitution will be given one of these handsome medals."

It was engraved with the image of a family—a man, woman and child—triumphantly holding a flaming torch aloft. The trio was encircled by the words: *Yea, I have a goodly heritage.* Returning the medallion to the girl, Tillie said, "It's heavier than it looks."

The girl stowed the medal in her pocket, then glanced at her clipboard. "Each participant is ranked on mental, physical and moral health based on the following criteria: your education; your occupation; any special talents, gifts, tastes or superior qualities; any serious illnesses you've suffered; any physical, mental or temperamental defects.

"All entrants must also submit blood and urine samples, have their height and weight measured, take an IQ test, and complete a questionnaire about their daily habits, medical history and social behaviour. Once your results are logged, you'll receive a letter grade to determine your eligibility for an award."

"A grade?" Tillie asked. "Like a teacher gives in school?"

"Sort of," the girl replied, showing Tillie a parchment certificate.

This is to certify that _____ has passed the Fitter Families Examination at the Michigan State Fair, August, 1930, and is entitled to be classified as _____ grade.

Signed _____

A gold foil seal graced the bottom corner of the document. *Like the grades meatpackers give to carcasses at the stockyard.*

"It's a simple, straightforward process that takes about three hours to complete."

"No, thank you," Tillie said. "I'm not interested."

She went to find Samuel, who was carrying paperwork of his own. "Henry Ford is looking for farmers to grow soybeans for him. Says he'll pay top dollar."

"What's Mr. Ford going to do with a bunch of soybeans?"

"Turn 'em into car parts."

"Car parts?"

"Yes. Soybeans into car parts. Imagine that."

Staring in the mirror, Tillie checks for other signs of her inevitable demise. She pats the soft skin under her chin with the back of her hand. Fifty-five. How will I know how to live?

The world has changed radically since she was young, since the days she trailed after her eldest brother in the barnyard, begging him to take her to the fair. Things she once thought astonishing are now commonplace—moving pictures, telephones, wireless radios, Mr. Ford's motorcars, women casting votes.

Sadly, the grief that has been so commonplace throughout her life has proved that it can still provide cruel astonishment. At the tender age of twenty, her eldest son, Charles, had taken ill and been admitted to the hospital, not with cancer but with a raging ear infection that led to a deadly brain abscess. The doctors performed emergency surgery, but within hours of the operation, he was gone. *Three years ago, this May.*

The rest of her children have stayed healthy, and all but two have left home. Her eldest, Katherine, has a child of her own, a baby girl.

The joy Tillie feels when holding her grandchild is bittersweet. Nothing can dispel the sadness she feels over the fact that her own mother never had the chance to do the same with her little ones.

Daughter number two, Grace, was married last summer, and daughter number three, Doris, will be next.

When Doris got engaged, Tillie had asked, "Have you set a date?"

"We're hoping for late June, in the back garden at the house, under the pergola, when the roses are in bloom. Nothing big. Just family and a few close friends," Doris replied.

Tillie wasn't surprised that Doris had already thought things through. She'd always been a mindful and observant child.

"And what about a dress?"

"Grace says I can wear hers."

"Is that what you want?"

"Yes. It's a perfect fit."

Tillie had secretly hoped that it might be daughter number four, Alice, who'd settle down next. Alice was just as intelligent and quick-witted as the rest of her siblings, but she was also eager to gossip, loose with the truth and prone to hold grudges. She'd been caught up with the same young man for some time now, and there'd been plenty of talk (between her sisters and around town) of secret meetings and late night trips to speakeasies in Detroit.

"Are you staying out of trouble?" she'd asked Alice, one rare evening when she was home for the night. "You're not keeping anything from me, are you?"

Alice had flashed the same impish grin she'd put on as a child whenever she'd gotten into mischief. "Why on earth would you think that?"

The pain in Tillie's belly clutches at her again, this time sharper, stronger, longer. Something's wrong. Something's there that shouldn't be.

She hears a voice whisper, "Deep inside, where life begins." Pauline had never been afraid to say what was on her mind or to confess her "knowings."

"I'm scared," Tillie says to her sister's ghost.

"Good."

"I don't want this."

"Who does?"

"Am I making something of nothing?"

"Make them listen. Insist."

"What if I'm wrong?"

"Do you think you are?"

"I'd like to be."

"That's not what I asked."

4087-AI   MATILDA WHEELER   4-3-31
                              Saline, Mich.

GYN: #24994. Age 54. Female. Domestic.

Hist: 3-4 attacks of slight vaginal bleeding during past year.

Dr. Brinkman. D&C Pathology

P.D.: Well advanced adenocarcinoma of endometrium,
becoming medullary.

The diagnosis comes quickly: *cancer of the uterus.*

The surgeon, Dr. Pierce, an associate professor at the university hospital, is direct. "We'll need to operate as soon as possible. I've scheduled a hysterectomy on the eighth. The sooner we get you in here, the better the chances."

"For?"

"Removing all the cancer."

"And after that?"

"We'll know once the surgery is over."

"Let's hope for the best, then."

"I see no reason why you shouldn't."

Tillie goes home, and tells O.C. She makes a few lists, packs a bag. Everything—their conversation, O.C.'s reaction, the doctor's plans, the course of her care, is matter of fact. O.C. reassures her (and himself) with talk of medical advances. She's frightened, but she can't bring herself to voice her fears. It feels important not to, as if doing so might cause the disease to react the same way dogs and horses do to nerves. She doesn't want to spook it, to risk it running wild.

The world has changed.

The astounding is now commonplace.

I must hope for the best.

Easter Sunday, when everyone is home for the holiday, she gives the girls and Bud the news. After answering their questions as best she can, she takes her new grandchild in her arms and steals away to the parlour. Settling in a rocking chair, she looks down at the sleepy-faced babe and smiles. "Keep your nose clean," she tells her. She refuses to say goodbye.

5078-AI MATILDA WHEELER 4-8-31

GYN: #248994. Age 54. Domestic. Hist: Vaginal bleeding.
Previous report on D&C by you was adenocarcinoma. Dr. Pierce.
Pan hysterectomy. Extent of the neoplasm? Prognosis? (8ss) See
16607-AI 4987-AI 371-AL 551-AU
P.D. : Atrophic ovaries with hyaline corpora fibrosa. Leiomyoma
in uterine wall. Chronic fibroid salpingitis. Recent partial curettage. Area of recent adenocarcinoma in endometrium, but no deep
invasion of myonobrrium in the area examined. Although farther
advanced . . . the prognosis should still be good. Cystic cervical
glands. CVW

Unlike every person in her family who'd had cancer before her, Tillie not only survives surgery—she lives.

SMITH-WHEELER

In the garden of the O.C. Wheeler home, Sunday, June 28 at 4 o'clock, Doris Martha, daughter of Mr. and Mrs. Wheeler, became the bride of Edward A. Smith of Indianapolis, Indiana. Reverend S. Schofield of the Methodist church performed the ceremony. The bride and her attendants in the lovely garden, created a picture of unusual beauty.

Miss Wheeler was given away in marriage by her father, before the pergola at the rear of the garden. Pink rambler roses and honeysuckle formed the background. The bride wore a gown of eggshell taffeta fashioned on simple lines. It was the gown worn by her sister at her marriage a year ago. A loose cap fastened with white rosebuds, lace mitts and kid pumps completed her costume. She carried an arm bouquet of talisman and white roses.

Immediately after the ceremony the guests retired to the house for a reception, which was decorated by the bride's mother with flowers from her garden.

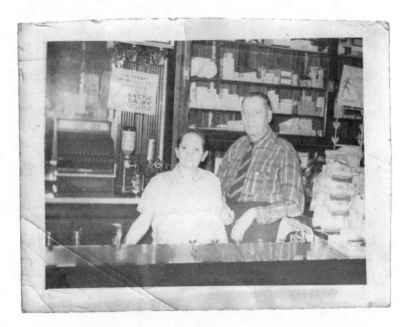

Tillie and O.C. at Wheeler's Drugs, circa 1944

21.

Thanksgiving

Lebanon, Indiana, 1992

Late November turns cold. The trees are already bare. My gut is constantly queasy. The next round of grad school exams is less than two weeks away and, in addition to dealing with my course work, I've been teaching an undergrad music theory class. I've also been trying to wrap my head around the fact that my advisor has left town to take a position at a school on the west coast. She'd been the only faculty member qualified to sign off on a thesis in musicology, so now I have to fend for myself until the music department can hire another musicologist to replace her. I've been informed that the faculty search will take at least a year, but I've only got one more semester's worth of classes before I'll need to settle on a topic for my thesis. Unless I transfer to another school or change my major, I'm stuck. On top of all that, I'd recently decided to shack up with my boyfriend. *Why not?* I'd thought. *Nothing else in my life is going as planned.*

I head home to my parents' for Thanksgiving, hoping for a reprieve from all my crap. Hanging out with Mom in the kitchen has always been good for what ails me.

"How's Ryan?" she asks as she brushes past me with a towering stack of Tupperware containers, ready to tackle post-Thanksgiving dinner cleanup.

Plucking the topmost container from the stack, I settle on a wooden stool at the kitchen counter. I'd volunteered to pick the remaining meat off the bones of the turkey. "It's not Ryan, Mom, it's Brian . . . and he's fine."

She sets the rest of the containers on the counter and begins to assess the leftovers. Her spatial acuity is pure witchery. Growing up I'd watched her fit all manner of unwieldy stuff into fridges, freezers, car trunks and closets. In my eyes, such talent is on par with watching David Copperfield make the Statue of Liberty disappear. Deftly scooping a heaping mound of mashed potatoes from a Dutch oven she adds, "You two settling in okay?"

Sorting white meat from dark, I answer, "We're doing all right."

The house Brian and I share with two of our classmates is a shabby little shotgun from the early 1900s just large enough for a quartet of struggling musicians and all our instruments: two French horns, a stand-up bass, a sousaphone, an electric bass, three flutes, a viola, a clarinet, a clunky upright piano and four trumpets in various states of repair. Brian's dad had bought the property with the understanding that we'd pay whatever rent we could afford each month. We'd been furnishing it with grungy finds from the Salvation Army, and had decorated the walls with half-finished expressionist studies we'd found in a dumpster behind the art department.

"Is there enough quiet in that place to get your work done?" Mom presses.

That place. She'd adored the last apartment I'd had, a sunny one-bedroom with high ceilings in a sprawling old Victorian house on the other side of town. Moving in with Brian had seemed a step backwards to her and she hadn't been shy about telling me so.

"It's fine," I reply, wiping glistening turkey fat from my fingers. "I can always go to my office at the university when I need to focus."

Mom pops a lid on the remains of the green bean casserole with a tight, final *snap.* "Right." Her skepticism is disturbingly well placed.

Living with Brian hadn't turned out to be as rosy as I'd hoped. When his schedule was loose, he was relaxed and fun. But when his schoolwork piled up (which was more often than not), he would spiral into a foul mood that was unpredictable and occasionally violent.

Two weeks before the break, I'd been paid to turn pages for Brian's accompanist at a French horn recital. Brian had performed brilliantly until partway through the last movement of his final piece when he'd hit a wrong note. It was a small mistake, something only another brass player might catch—a slight whiff, a blip, a frack. Although he'd easily finished the piece, he couldn't let the slip go. After taking an awkward bow, he'd stormed off the stage, cursing, and run to the green room. I'd watched in disbelief as he'd thrown his horn to the floor and kicked it into a crumpled mess. The angry clatter of the instrument's bell against the linoleum stopped me in my tracks. Our horn instructor, a soft-spoken man we affectionately called "Doc," had taken my arm and gently said, "Go home. I'll take care of this." The next morning I'd gotten out of bed to find Brian passed out on the couch, a borrowed horn in a new case at his side. When I'd finally worked up the courage to ask him about the incident, he'd given me a helpless shrug. "I messed up," he said.

"You want to talk about it?"

"Nope."

That was that.

I'd studied music long enough to know this sort of behaviour wasn't unusual in our profession. Beethoven was a cranky, dirty slob. Mussorgsky drank himself to death. Mozart was a foul-mouthed brat. Robert Schumann suffered from mental breakdowns so often that his wife, Clara (herself a fine composer and pianist), took on managing the house and earning an income while raising their seven kids. Music history was rife with tortured souls and complex characters, which was the main reason I was drawn to study it.

The circle Brian and I currently ran in had its share of drama. Many musicians at the university freely passed around prescription meds to stifle anxiety and stage fright. Others stuck to booze, pot and other illicit drugs. Most added a good deal of sex to the mix. If you were in the music department, you were bound to get tangled up in some (or all) of it. I'd done a decent job of sticking close to my books and scores, but over the past year Brian and I had consistently wound up together at parties, after rehearsals, and in practice rooms at 3:00 a.m. I'd thought living together would keep us sane and away from other people's messes.

"Is it serious?" Mom asks, now turning her attention to the dirty china on the dining-room table.

"Is what serious?"

"Your thing with Brian."

"I don't know," I say, packing up the turkey and washing my hands.

"Too soon to tell?"

"Too soon for you to ask."

I desperately wanted whatever was happening between Brian and me to be love, to have a relationship like the one my parents had. That was supposed to be the goal, right? I'd be the Clara to Brian's Robert, if that's what it took. I'd hold back his darkness with my light.

Mom puts her hand on the small of my back. "Are you feeling all right? You seem a little out of sorts."

"I'm just tired," I say. "School's been busy." Smiling, I pat my belly. "Or maybe I just ate too much."

We laugh.

She backs off, for now.

I can't help but think that I should be worrying over her, instead of the other way around. She'd spent the last three days preparing a feast for thirteen people that'd taken less than an hour to consume. It'd been just over a year since her surgery and chemo, and only recently had she gotten back to her fighting weight. "No more bag o' bones," she'd proudly declared.

But her life continued to be an endless stream of medical tests, doctor appointments and waiting to get the "all clear." She'd embraced the holiday with fervour, controlling every aspect of the meal. I'd helped as much as she'd allowed me to, but mostly I'd stayed out of her way. She'd come out the other side of her cancer sinewy, cheeky, tough.

"How about you let me finish up here," I say, looking at the piles of dishes she's lined up on the counter. The china, Noritake Blue Hill, had been a gift from my father for their thirtieth anniversary. They'd eloped the summer of '54 just after his tour of duty in Japan had ended, so there'd been no registry, no fancy dress, no wedding china. Even though her dishwasher has a delicate cycle, she insists on washing each plate by hand. "Go have a rest," I say, but it falls on deaf ears.

She runs warm water in the left side of the stainless steel sink and squeezes dish soap onto a rag. A few stray bubbles float into the air and dance around her face as she gestures to the linen drawer with her sponge. "I'll wash, you dry."

I tried.

"How's Alice?" I ask as I take the first wet salad plate in hand.

"Holding her own," Mom replies, searching the soapy water for another plate.

It'd been a couple of years since my grandmother had been to our house for Thanksgiving. I missed helping her bake yeast rolls and opening tiny cans of mandarin oranges for her ambrosia salad. I wasn't sure if this year's absence was due to her own aches and pains or if Mom's cancer had been too much for her to take. "Did she have any plans for today?"

"I think she stayed at the nursing home for dinner, or maybe she went to your aunt's? You should go see her sometime. Take that boyfriend of yours with you. She'd like that."

I feel as if I should apply Mom's advice more to visiting her than Alice. Between schoolwork and the move and my own inability to deal with her illness, I've become increasingly absent from her life the last few months. Since she never complained about her struggles or asked me for anything, I kept at my work and told myself she was going to be fine.

Dry plate in hand, I open the cupboard where Mom keeps the good china. These days it's also a repository for all her insurance forms and medical paperwork. Countless prescriptions and appointment reminders flank the cups and saucers. Mom calls over her shoulder, "Don't forget the coffee filters." It's a hard and fast rule: The dishes aren't to be put away without a filter between each plate.

As I put the salad dishes away in order, I notice a bright pink slip marked "copy" tacked to the inside of the cupboard door.

PERMISSION FORM

I hereby agree to permit the Department of Preventive
Medicine at Creighton University and the Hereditary Cancer

Consultation Center to obtain my medical records, pathology
slides and tissue blocks from attending physicians and hospitals,
in furtherance of the research studies they are conducting.

"What's this?" I ask, pointing to the paper.

"Didn't I tell you? I got a call from Dr. Lynch."

"Who?"

"Henry Lynch, the doctor in Nebraska who's been keeping tabs
on the family all these years. I let him know about my cancer and he
asked if he could have my records."

"And your tissues?" This was all sounding a bit too Frankenstein
for me.

"Yes, from my tumour and a sample of my blood too."

"What's he going to do with it?"

"He hopes it'll help researchers crack the code to the family's
cancer."

"Really?"

"He says they're getting closer every day."

After Aldred Warthin's death in 1931, his assistant, Carl Weller, had
carried on with the study of Family G. Weller and his colleagues continued to trace the cancer-status of family members for some time, but
with the shadow of Warthin's eugenics-based theories looming and no
real answers surfacing, the family's participation eventually waned.

Warthin's research and the family's medical records languished in
a dark closet in the university's pathology department for nearly three
decades until Henry Lynch came on the scene. Determined to prove
that a genetic link to certain cancers did exist, Dr. Lynch forged his
own relationship with a new generation of Family G members in the
mid-1960s. Mom had been a fan ever since.

My memories of the man we called "Dr. Henry" had come from
a family cancer register that Mom kept safely tucked away in the
bottom drawer of her dresser. The first time I'd seen it was when I was
in Grade 2 and my class had been assigned to create a family tree
for the US bicentennial. The other kids had brought in stories of

ancestors who'd fought in wars or held political office. (It seemed like half the class was related to George Washington.) The instant Mom had shown me the register with its foldout pedigree charts and its long lists of dates and names, I was enthralled. The brown paper cover featured two remarkable images: a hazy portrait of a family dressed in Victorian garb, and a drawing of a rustic homestead with barn and windmill. *The Family G Register*, by Anne Krush and Henry T. Lynch. For the longest time, I believed that Anne and Henry were family too. How could these researchers my mother revered not be kin?

"What does getting closer mean?" I ask, plucking an envelope from Creighton U. out of the cabinet.

"Hopefully that one day there'll be no more cancer." She nods her permission for me to read the letter.

> At Creighton University we study the way cancers or tumors occur in a family by collecting a detailed medical history, then drawing a family tree. Any pattern that appears will help us decide if a family has an increased risk of cancer due to genetic factors, and may even help us identify individuals who are at high genetic risk of having cancer.

"You know I'd said to myself if I got through this damn mess that I wouldn't waste any more time. Dr. Lynch is giving me a chance to do something big. This could help not just our family, but others too. We have to do our part."

I put the letter back in its place and go to her side. "I'm proud of you, Mom."

"Thanks, kiddo."

She holds out the gravy boat for me to dry, but when I go to take it from her, it slips out of my hand and crashes against the edge of the sink. Hunks of china go flying.

"Oh, God, Mom," I say, gathering broken pieces in the palm of my hand. It can't be repaired. "I'm so sorry!"

"It's all right," she says, surveying the damage. "You didn't cut yourself, did you?"

"No," I say, and I burst into tears.

Mom takes the shards of china from me and wraps them in paper towel before she tucks them in the garbage.

"You waited so long for that china," I sob. "And now it's ruined."

"We can get another gravy boat . . ."

"You work so hard, Mom, and I fucked it all up."

"Language, sweetie. Heavens—it's just a thing." Giving me a hug, she says, "Is there something you want to tell me?"

"No," I answer. "I'm fine."

I spend the next week puking my guts up every morning before class. Friday afternoon, I walk to the drugstore and buy a pregnancy test, then go to the women's bathroom of the Fine Arts building and pee on a little plastic stick. After carefully transporting the stick to my office, I lay it on top of my desk. The shelves beside the desk hold music by Mozart, Berlioz, Copland, Barber, Beethoven, Schubert, Bach. There's a copy of Clara Schumann's Nocturne tucked somewhere among them. She wrote it when she was seventeen, when she was still Clara Wieck. At 90 bpm, andante con moto, it takes five minutes to play, two minutes longer than it takes a pregnancy test to sort itself out.

I watch the window on the stick and wait. If you look closely you can see the change happen, a shadow crossing left to right, leaving a little mark in its wake.

+

22.

For Auld Lang Syne

Nova Scotia, December 31, 2017
New Year's Eve. 11:00 p.m. AST.

I'm curled on the couch in front of the TV with my husband and youngest son, trying not to fall asleep. Earlier in the evening we'd played a few board games and polished off what remained of the Christmas sweets. Now we're flipping channels—cruising between old movies, local news, and the latest footage from Times Square. I have a hard time not worrying that something terrible will happen to the people gathered there. This is the world in which we live, the only one my youngest son has ever known. I can't watch the sea of revellers jostling, cheering, dancing in place, without thinking that gunfire, or a bomb, or someone driving a truck into the crowd won't suddenly shatter their joy. How many times can things like that happen before we're irrevocably broken? Maybe we already are. Am I alone in thinking this? I don't mention it. I don't want to spoil the quiet, sleepy closeness of the moment: we three huddled together in a little room at the top of our little house in our little corner of the planet as the TV casts a flickering glow over us.

Anderson Cooper says it's the coldest New Year's Eve in a century, the second coldest on record for Times Square. I believe it. The poor guy looks frozen to the bone. "Why isn't he wearing a hat?" I ask, channelling my mom. "Would someone get him some earmuffs, or a toque already? His ears are bright red."

My son laughs. He's knitting a hat. His fourth this month.

Anderson tells us that a few brave souls arrived as early as 7:00 a.m. to stake out prime locations for viewing the ball drop. I detected a hint of "if you think I'm nuts, then get a load of this" in his voice as he'd said it, which leads me to wonder if he'd somehow heard the collective sigh of mothers around the globe over his lack of proper headwear. Anderson's frost-nipped ears aside, I marvel at the fact that despite the frigid conditions and the spectres of terrors past, people have gathered in droves to stand together to cheer and sing and kiss and ring in the New Year. One hundred thousand of them. I look at their half-frozen faces and goofy hats and think, *I don't have what it takes to do that.*

It also occurs to me that I've got absolutely no desire to make resolutions this year. There are too many loose ends in my life—looming deadlines, my eldest son's genetic testing, my not-yet-scheduled annual colonoscopy, a heart monitor test booked for mid-January. I'd spent the past week living in the magical bubble of days between Christmas and the New Year, all responsibilities forgotten. Now the clock is ticking fast towards midnight and all the lebkuchen is gone. Maybe if I fall asleep before twelve, the New Year will never come. Maybe all the sugar from the cookies has gone to my head. Maybe I'm just getting old.

When I was a kid, my whole family stayed home on New Year's Eve. We'd spin LPs on my Dad's hi-fi or turn on *Dick Clark's New Year's Rockin' Eve* while we devoured pretzels and chips, and played round after round of whoop-tee-do and zilch. As midnight approached, the snacks, cards and dice were set aside so we could gather in the backyard to light leftover sparklers from the Fourth of July and watch Dad shoot his trusty .22 into the starry night. Once the celebratory *crack!* of the rifle had sounded, we'd troop inside to witness Mom popping open a bottle of Martini & Rossi. Scrambling around the room, I'd search under the coffee table, behind the stereo cabinet and between couch cushions, believing that if I retrieved the shot cork, I'd gain enough luck to last the whole year.

※

At 11:20 p.m. AST I send a group text to my brothers and sister. Nova Scotia is an hour ahead of where they are and I doubt I'll make it to midnight EST.

> **Me:** Happy New Year!!! In case I fall asleep . . .
> **Doug:** Happy New Year everybody!
> **Lori:** happy new year. love you all and best wishes. 🙏

My eldest brother, Skip, is out with friends. His response will come tomorrow morning along with a video of an Australian shepherd who likes to go tobogganing.

My siblings and I aren't in touch often, and I see them even less. When Mom was alive, we funnelled all our news through her, knowing she'd pass the important bits and pieces on to the rest of the family. At the time it'd seemed efficient, prudent, right. After she died, we relied on Dad to broadcast the news of our lives, but now that we've lost him too, we've had to learn to navigate our communications on our own, hoping that our blood ties will see us through to a new way of connecting. I fear that our attempts at closeness will always be a work in progress.

Most of our conversations begin by one of us apologizing for how long it's been since they last called. Lori firmly believes it doesn't matter if it's been two days, six weeks or twelve months because, she says, "We have the kind of connection that allows us to pick up where we left off." I want to believe that's true, and most of the time it is, but lately it feels as if the distance is too great and there's too much to explain, especially when it comes to the intense self-examination I've chosen to undertake by writing about Lynch syndrome. The last thing I want is to burden them with any of it. Both of my brothers have had cancer, and my sister, although free from Lynch syndrome, has recently been diagnosed with MS. They have their own families, lives, aches and pains. I assume they've already worked through their shit and don't need to hear mine. Besides, I've always had a tendency to get deep, existential and weird, fast. As a child I could easily spend thirty minutes describing the path I'd seen a ladybug take to get from one leaf to another. Such tales often included klutzy hand gestures and spilled milk, along with a series of increasingly angst-ridden questions based on information I'd gleaned from nursery rhymes and fairy tales. "Was her house on fire? Were her children burning?" My siblings sometimes snickered over my dinner-table dramatics, but if they saw I was in true distress, they always came to my aid. Why, then, am I so afraid to tell them of my fears surrounding cancer, and the things we share through our DNA?

I'm fearful they still see me as a child, or worse, as weak and self-absorbed. I'm afraid they'll simply tell me to "stop worrying." That was their M.O. when I was little. Now that we're adults, all I really want is for at least one of them to say that sometimes they get scared too.

By the end of January, Mom will have been gone eleven years. By mid-April, Dad will have been gone for six. I have no idea who currently lives in the house where I grew up. My friend Dawn passes by the place every so often and reports back to me its condition. She always says it looks fine. I wouldn't want to know if it didn't. In my heart it's forever spring on Perry-Worth Road, and Mom's daffodils are nodding their sunny yellow heads along the driveway as the magnolia in the front yard eternally reaches for the sky.

I lived in that house from the day I was born until I left for university just after my eighteenth birthday. Money was tight then, and phone calls were expensive. Knowing my tendency to ramble, Mom had come up with a code. "If you're out late or missing home, call and let the phone ring once and hang up. I'll do the same in reply." From me it meant: *I made it back. I'm safe.* From her: *I love you.* Long after the number had been disconnected, I'd still pick up the phone and dial home. Sometimes I still do.

11:59 p.m. AST. My cell phone dings. It's my eldest son in Halifax.

Eldest Son: One minute!!!
Me: Woohoo! We're all still awake!
Eldest Son: 4, 3 . . .
Me: . . . 2, 1!
Eldest Son: 🎆 🎆 🎆

I exchange kisses with my husband, then hug Youngest Son (and silently rejoice that the wry, brilliant lad still puts up with me hugging him).

"Happy New Year!"

"Woohoo!"

"Here's to 2018!"

Turning back to my phone, I text Eldest Son.

Me: Happy New year, kiddo!!

Eldest Son: Happy New Year!! Love you! HFITM!

Me: Love you too! HFITM!

HFITM—"Happy face in the morning!"—our signature farewell, and what my mom and I always said to each other at the end of every phone call.

Youngest Son scoops up his knitting needles and yarn and heads off to bed. Ian takes the dog outside for a New Year's pee. I go downstairs to check the fire. As I stir the coals, Ian knocks on the door, three pieces of firewood tucked under his arm, asking to be let in. The dog barks at his odd behaviour, mistaking Ian's "first-foot" as a plea for help rather than a tradition passed down from his ancestors.

I let them both inside, then wipe snow from the dog's paws as Ian tends the fire.

We go upstairs, brush our teeth, tuck into bed.

As I'm drifting off to sleep, I hear a coyote let go a long, melancholy howl. "Do you hear that?" I ask, giving Ian a soft but urgent nudge.

"Hmm?" he replies, rolling over and finding my hand. After eighteen years of marriage, he's experienced enough of my late-night writing jags and oddball revelations to know there's no reason to panic.

"I think I heard a coyote . . . close, between the house and the barn."

He reaches over and opens the window a couple of inches. Cold air rushes in. We curl together under the covers and listen.

The animal howls again, then waits.

There's no answer. No reply.

"She's alone," I whisper, my heart breaking for her in the silence.

The coyote calls again, this time punctuating her cry with a string of plaintive yips.

Each time she howls, I feel more tender and raw.

Her song continues, echoing through mossy spruce, as my husband's breathing slows and he falls asleep.

The longer she howls, the more I'm tempted to run downstairs and howl to her off the back porch. I want to give her the response she desires, but I'm not her kind. The differences between us are too great, our connection, too tenuous. I can never be what she needs.

After the longest cry yet, she moves on, her howls growing ever more distant as she makes her way back into the woods.

Closing the window, I whisper to my husband, "Happy New Year, my love."

As I lay my head on my pillow, he rouses enough to plant a sleepy kiss on my cheek.

I am not alone.

23

Three Hundred and Five

Boston, Massachusetts, 1936
On a crisp clear morning in April, two days before Good Friday, doctors, researchers and educators gather at Harvard University for the twenty-ninth annual meeting of the American Association for Cancer Research. One by one, the attendees—from universities, hospitals, private laboratories and pharmaceutical companies across the US—walk across the grassy courtyard, pass between the Doric columns of Peter Bent Brigham Hospital, enter the light-filled vestibule, and carry on into the hospital's storied amphitheatre.

Among the day's presenters is Dr. Carl Weller from the University of Michigan. The clean-cut forty-nine-year-old pathologist with round spectacles and a dimpled chin is there with his colleague I.J. Hauser to deliver "A Further Report on the Cancer Family of Warthin." Weller had studied under Aldred Warthin, and then gone on to collaborate with him on several projects, including Family G. When Warthin died in 1931, Weller had been awarded the position of director of pathological laboratories and been given the go-ahead to continue with Warthin's research.

Now, as Weller waits to take his place at the lectern, he thinks through the points of his presentation one last time. He's keenly aware of the resistance Warthin faced from the association in the past—the battle between those who preferred to look at extrinsic factors as the cause of cancer versus those who were convinced heredity played a key role. When it comes to Warthin's work, many questions and doubts remain. Weller also knows that he's less stubborn and brash than his predecessor, and less inclined to eugenics. He prefers to keep his head down and do the work of compiling facts and figures, believing that the data will provide a path to something more than they have now. He has already seen great changes occur—in his lab, in the hospital and in Family G.

And so, two decades after a seamstress confided her fears to Aldred Warthin, Weller delivers an address to the country's leading cancer researchers on the state of her kin. No family members are present, but they're never far from his mind. He's met with many of them over the years, crossed paths with them in the corridors of University Hospital, made tissue blocks and slides from their diseased flesh.

He begins. "The family with numerous deaths from cancer, which was reported by Dr. A.S. Warthin in 1913 and 1925, has been referred to wherever the intrinsic factor of the aetiology of malignancy has been discussed. Now that twenty-three years have passed since the first study of this family, it is appropriate again to bring its history up to date. This large group now consists of six generations and three hundred and five individuals."

Weller's opening salvo also includes the declaration of a "cancer age" for the family of "twenty-five years," determined by the earliest age of occurrence. "The average age at which cancer has been diagnosed in this family, or at which death from cancer has occurred, as the case may be, is forty-eight point three years." Overall, the development of malignant neoplasms in the family is at an incidence rate of 27.5 percent.

As he presents an overview of each branch of the family, Weller illustrates the most prominent cancer cases with a series of lantern slides he's chosen from the hundreds of tissue samples the laboratory has collected over the years: adenocarcinoma of the endometrium, gland-cell carcinoma of the cecum, adenocarcinoma of the descending colon, adenocarcinoma of the rectum. "The anatomical distribution of cancer within this family presents one of its most interesting features. The gastrointestinal tract and the uterus are primary sites."

Within the pages of the report, each case has been assigned an alphanumeric code, according to an identification system Warthin devised when he first began his study of the family. Weller, of course, also knows every person behind each case by name—Rosa, age forty-two; Ida, age forty-one; Peter, age fifty-two; Pauline, age forty-six; Tillie, age fifty-five . . . all of them, except one, are now deceased. The deaths that had hit him the hardest among the members of Family G had come the year before Pauline Gross died, when two young male relatives had been admitted to the hospital for appendicitis on the same day, then both found to have inoperable cancer. Ruben, age thirty; Elmer, age twenty-seven. At Warthin's behest, Weller had been assigned to perform their autopsies.

"To date, fifteen cancerous individuals have died without off-spring—ten male, five female. Nine of the men and four of the women did not marry." He doesn't say that they'd likely taken Warthin's lectures on the taint in their blood to heart, but he does mention that if members of the family don't reproduce, there is less cancer.

In addition to this, he points out that although two branches seem to be free of the disease and that the incidence of cancer may be decreasing in the younger generations, "this may be more apparent than real. Not until the full effect of age becomes known in respect to the third and fourth generations can this be determined."

Declaring "Branch K"—Pauline's maternal line—as "highly cancerous," he explains that, even so, a member of that branch, "the sixth child of K, a daughter," is living despite having developed two primary carcinomas. The seamstress's sister, Tillie, is the first in the family to survive cancer. Not only that, but she's done so twice.

"In 1931," Weller reads, "panhysterectomy was done for a well-advanced adenocarcinoma of the endometrium. In 1933 the cecum was resected for an extensive fungating adenocarcinoma of a quite different nature." Tillie's first cancer had been Warthin's final Family G case, but the man who'd once called her family inferior stock hadn't lived long enough to witness her astounding strength and persistence. Both times, she'd come to the hospital when the first signs of disease had presented themselves and insisted upon seeing a surgeon. She's a grandmother four times over now. Three circles and one square on that chart of 305. Weller doesn't mention this. Instead, he concludes with what he hopes is now a self-evident proposition: "This family provides very strong presumptive evidence for an inheritable organ-specific predisposition to carcinoma."

As he waits for questions from the floor, the audience shifts in their seats. Men of science have been arguing in this hall since 1913, the year Warthin first introduced Family G to the medical literature.

The first query comes from the conference chair, Dr. E.T. Bell, who stands and asks, "I should like to know if the extent to which cancer persists in this family after intermarriage with other presumably non-cancerous families indicates any dominant influence in heredity."

Before Weller can answer, Dr. C.C. Little intervenes. The two men aren't strangers. Clarence Cook Little had served as the president of the University of Michigan from 1925 to 1929, and had also served as president of the American Eugenics Society. After leaving the university, he'd opened his own lab at the University of Maine in Bar Harbor, Maine—an epicentre of eugenics research—with funding from some of the wealthiest supporters of the movement. These days Little mostly deals in genetic experimentation with mice, but the subject of heredity as applied to the human species is always foremost in his mind. While in Ann Arbor, he'd run in the same circles as Warthin, often enlisting the pathologist to speak at various gatherings in order to spread the gospel of race betterment.

Broad-chested and well-dressed, the former captain of the Harvard track team is an imposing figure, even from a distance. "It seems to me that this study is extremely important," he says, "and that Dr. Warthin in starting it, and Dr. Weller in continuing it, have done a real service. Is the level of intelligence in the family such that it appreciates that it is being studied as a cancer family, and will the younger people in the family tend to avoid intermarriage with other cancer families, as I know some younger people do, if their own family has a tendency in that direction?"

The thought that the family might be living according to eugenic principles clearly excites Little, but he knows better than to lay it out plainly. These are the ideas, after all, that have created the controversy that follows him everywhere he goes, flowing from the same philosophy that is fuelling the rise of Nazism in Germany. He's carefully couched his ideas in language that's palatable to the committee, but clear enough for sympathetic ears. A far cry from the speech he'd given as chair of the Third Race Betterment Conference of 1928 where he'd said: "Many people are born more or less defective, in one or another of their constitutional elements, and in the correction of these deficiencies we are making real advancements." That particular conference had boasted such lectures as: "The Menace of the Melting Pot," "Who Outbreeds Whom?" and "Race Deterioration and Destruction with Special Reference to the American People." It was the same forum where Warthin had first introduced his infamous "biological creed."

Rather than giving Weller a chance to answer, Little holds the floor. "I feel that there may be a very interesting chance in this family, even if we cannot find any definite law of inheritance, to be on the lookout for early cancer or precancerous conditions, and I know Dr. Weller's interest in cancer educational work is such as to make that a branch of the study which he has planned."

It sounds innocent enough, possibly even progressive, but "education" in relation to Little's beloved eugenics is a slippery slope. Backed by funding from the Carnegie Institute, the Eugenics Record Office in Cold Springs, New York, has been actively compiling reports, articles, charts and pedigrees on family genetic traits for years. The information they've gathered, in the form of thousands of family files, is currently being used to support the practice of forced sterilizations. Little had worked at the Cold Springs lab before taking the position in Bar Harbor.

Weller is just about to respond, when Dr. James Ewing, current president of Memorial Hospital in New York, steps in. At seventy years of age, the lanky, unassuming pathologist is known as "the Chief" among his colleagues, and more recently, "Cancer Man Ewing," after being featured on the cover of *Time* magazine in 1931. Ewing's research primarily focuses on radiation treatments for cancer, so he's seen the worst that the disease can do to the human body. He's suspicious of Little's enthusiasm, and of anything that smells like agenda-based science. After thanking Weller for his "valuable service" in continuing work on Family G, the old man cuts to the chase: "I have never been able . . . to become enthusiastic over the subject of cancer families.

Dr. Warthin undoubtedly encountered a family in which cancer was unusually frequent, but we should remember that people inherit the living quarters, the habits, and even the old clothes of their forebears, as well as their physical constitution, and I cannot see . . . adequate grounds for assuming that inheritance was really of a general cancer tendency."

Point by point, he proceeds to pull Weller's research apart, pointing out what he describes as "many sources of statistical error," mostly in an effort to push back against Little. Then, in a direct admonishment of Little, he adds, "Dr. Weller does not attempt to draw any definite conclusions from the newly reported data, and probably none can be drawn at present."

When, at last, Weller takes his turn, he does his best to address the concerns of both men.

"In answer to Dr. Little's question: I think many of the things he brought out are actually occurring in the family; not that they are deliberately avoiding intermarriage with other cancer families, for I think they would seldom have knowledge of prevalent cancer in other lines, but there is no doubt that some members of the family are avoiding marriage and offspring. There is a deliberate attempt in certain branches of the family to bring the family line to a close.

"Also, these cancers are being diagnosed earlier than in previous years. Most of the members of this family will consult a doctor for degrees of indigestion that would probably not lead the average individual to seek medical advice."

Turning to Ewing, he says: "I appreciate very much Dr. Ewing's critical analysis of the situation. I invite attention to the fact that the larger the family gets, the less is the element of chance in connection with the statistics which it includes. The larger the family gets, the more sure we will be as to the significance of any deviation, one way or another, in its general behaviour as compared to the population as a whole." After reiterating the ways in which the family's cancers are "not behaving according to the general statistical expectation," he concludes, "this family exhibits a strong genetic peculiarity in its susceptibility to cancer."

In early August 1936, Time magazine publishes an account of these events, which in turn is then printed in newspapers across the US. Its text is laced with ominous phrases and dire predictions.

CANCER STRIKES 6 GENERATIONS
Malady Dogs Family Since 1856.

Long before the civil war a German known to medical history only as G settled in wild Washtenaw County, Michigan, near the village of Ann Arbor.

The fourth generation of this remarkable cancer family was breeding away when it came to the attention of the late Professor Aldred Scott Warthin.

All members of this family have good reason to fear being stricken by the age of 25.

It is the stuff of Tillie's nightmares. Her youngest grandchild is only two years of age—number 305 in Weller's study.

She will become my mother.

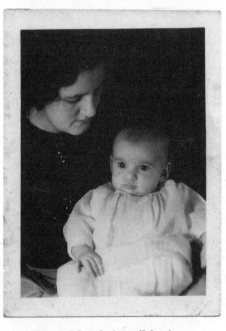

Alice and Sarah Anne (Mom), 1933

24.

Sarah Anne

Saline, Michigan, 1937

Tillie watches her grandchildren as they laugh and play in the garden behind her house. There are five of them now—the eldest is nine, the youngest, just shy of two months old.

The hot July day has turned into a family reunion of sorts, with all of Tillie and O.C.'s brood there to witness the christenings of the four youngest grandchildren. Doc is plopped in the grass, deep in conversation with the little ones. They've dubbed him their "waboo" and treat him as if he's their king.

As Tillie looks on, she thinks, *Wasn't it only yesterday that he was chasing Bud, Charles and the girls around the yard?*

Their four eldest have married and moved out of town: Kate to Midland, Grace to Dearborn, Doris to southern Indiana, and Alice, just a stone's throw away, to Plymouth.

She's glad Alice hasn't gone far. Although if anyone had told her that she'd ever think such a thing, she would've laughed and called them crazy. She and Alice had had their share of disagreements the last few years, mostly due to her daughter's fondness for bending the truth. The girl's biggest transgression thus far had come in the form of her elopement, which Alice had confessed to her mother, just after Doris's wedding. It turned out Alice had been secretly married for an entire year at that point.

"A year?" Tillie had put her hand to her mouth. "*Gott im Himmel.*"

The only times she spoke German anymore were while attending family funerals or when she wished to stifle a curse.

"We had no choice," Alice had insisted. "James's parents were against us from the start. They threatened to disown him if we wed."

Tillie didn't object to the union, even though James Mackintosh was the same young man Alice had reportedly been frequenting speakeasies with in Detroit. From what she could tell, he seemed like a steady enough lad, which was precisely what her daughter needed. "And you didn't think to come to your father and me? We could've spoken to his parents on your behalf."

"It wouldn't have helped." The Mackintoshes had roundly rejected not only Alice but her entire family, but she wasn't about to admit this to her mother.

"Why are you telling me this now?" Tillie pressed. "Are you with child?"

"No."

"Don't lie to me."

"I'm not." Alice insisted. "James's parents have finally come around. The only thing they ask is that we get married at St. Andrew's in Ann Arbor. I knew I couldn't ask for your blessing without being completely honest with you first."

"You think you can keep a secret like that from me, and still expect my blessing?"

"I'd hoped you'd understand."

An uneasy silence had fallen between them as Tillie sorted her thoughts. She was wounded, hurt, at a loss. It was all too easy for her to imagine James's parents' complaints about her daughter. *Not good enough. A poor match. Bad stock.*

"Please don't be angry, Mama," Alice had begged. "We did it for love."

Tillie wished that love could set everything right. "What is it that you want, Alice?"

"I want to do whatever it takes for them to accept me."

"Then I guess we'd better start planning a proper wedding."

☙

But that was then and this is now. Squeals of laughter erupt from across the lawn as O.C. scoops up Alice's daughter, Sarah Anne, in his arms and whirls her through the air. She is a blur of dark curls and ruffled petticoats. She'll turn four, come late August. When it comes down to it, this little girl is the reason why Tillie has finally been able to forgive Alice.

"Waboo!" the other children shout with glee. "Pick me! Pick me!"

Sarah Anne had been born the year that Tillie's eldest brother, Samuel, had taken ill with cancer and Tillie herself had been struck a second time. When Samuel had died and Tillie had survived, Tillie couldn't help but wonder why she was still alive. Of her nine siblings, only three remained. The birth of Alice's first child had been a gift, shaking her free from the compulsion to spend every waking minute interrogating God.

She'd looked after the little girl when Alice and James had decided to begin breeding cocker spaniels for show. The young couple had enthusiastically embraced the world of bloodlines and pedigrees, sires and dams, studs and bitches, travelling from city to city in pursuit of blue ribbons and silver trophies.

Tillie was the one who had seen Sarah Anne through teething and measles and learning to walk. In return, the sweet, curious child had given her a reason to get well, carry on, try harder.

With all her grandchildren in mind, she'd forged a relationship with Dr. Weller, supplying him with as much information as she could—who'd died, who'd gotten married, who'd had children, who'd fallen ill. Sadly, it didn't matter how much she told the doctor, or how much blood and flesh she gave the university, the constant, invasive questioning of her and her kin had led not to a cure or a solution but to reinforcing the notion that they were "an unfortunate family." Still she wouldn't give up, not yet.

She'd held Sarah Anne's first birthday in the garden surrounded by black-eyed Susans, garden phlox and hollyhocks in full bloom. The tiny cake she'd baked for the girl, decked with buttercream frosting and a single candle, had served as both a celebration of Sarah Anne's growth and a testament to Tillie's perseverance.

"Nana!" the child calls as O.C. brings her safely back to earth.

Tillie crouches and smiles and holds her arms out to her grand-daughter.

There's a light in the little girl's eyes that reminds her of Pauline. What she wouldn't give for the two of them to have met. She's certain Sarah Anne holds the same spark of determination as her sister, the same forthright spirit. Wrapping the child in a warm embrace, she wonders, *What can I give her to help her find her way?*

Truth.

Attention.

Hope.

Love.

Four grandchildren of Mr and Mrs O.C. Wheeler were christened at the family home on Sunday: Harold Wheeler Hilsinger, son of Mr and Mrs Harold Hilsinger of Midland; Suzanne Grace Smith, daughter of Mr and Mrs Edward Smith of Seymour, Indiana; Sarah Anne Mackintosh, daughter of Mr and Mrs James Mackintosh of Plymouth; and Genanne Jane Young, the infant daughter of Mr and Mrs C.J. Young of Dearborn.

Each of the granddaughters, including Marjorie Ann Hilsinger, has Anne as part of her name, after that of their grand-mother, Matilda Anne Wheeler.

The service was read at 3:30 by Rev. Andrew Kurth of Detroit.

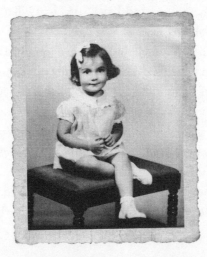

Mom at three

25.

Induction

Terre Haute, Indiana, 1993

My mother and I are sitting on a bench in the shady courtyard of St. Stephen's Episcopal Church.

"I'm scared, Mom. I'm really afraid."

"I know you are, honey, but you'll get through it."

I'd been coming to this quiet green space surrounded by shadowy alcoves and criss-crossed by stone walkways since my first year of university. Close to campus, it'd been the ideal spot to clear my head after long rehearsals and stressful exams. I'd never attended services there, but the courtyard had always provided me with solace and rest—two things I desperately need on this sweltering August day. I am two weeks overdue and I'd just been told to report to the hospital at 5:00 a.m. to have my labour induced.

Clutching my mom's hand I say, "This isn't what I had planned."

"It never is," she replies.

I half expect her to launch into her usual "on the day you were born" speech, the one in which she almost gleefully catalogues the harrowing details of my birth. As a kid, I'd loved hearing the play-by-play of that rainy July afternoon: *My regular doctor had gone on vacation, the emergency doc was an intern, he took one look between my legs and said "It's a girl." Breech births were really risky back then, we both could've died. . . .*

Thinking of it now makes me queasy.

But Mom reads my rattled mind. "What happened to me isn't what's going to happen to you. At least this kid is turned the right way around."

"Oh God is it ever," I say, willing my water to break right there on the spot. The baby and its bowling ball of a head have been dropped for what feels like an eternity. My bag's packed, the baby's room is finished, the car seat's been installed. It's the thought of being hooked up to a fetal monitor and an IV drip full of chemicals that's throwing me. "I wanted it to be natural, easy."

"Come on, now," Mom says. "I've never known you to do *anything* the easy way." Placing her hand on my belly she adds, "This baby's just stubborn, like you. You're both going to be fine."

When I'd first discovered I was pregnant, I kept the news to myself. For two agonizing weeks, I took multiple pregnancy tests while grappling with a list of daunting questions that relentlessly nagged in my head. Am I ready to be a mother? Is abortion the better choice? What if Brian doesn't want it? Can I raise a child on my own?

I had close friends who'd found themselves in the same situation—some had chosen to terminate their pregnancies, others now had babies in tow. Either way, their lives had been forever changed.

I'd always planned on having kids, *someday*. My sister had had her first child at eighteen. I was twenty-four. The more I thought about it, the more I found myself wanting this child more than anything I'd ever wanted in my life.

So I took on pregnancy the same way I'd tackled school, checking out armloads of books from the library, filling three-ring binders with handwritten notes. As a grad student, I couldn't afford to see an obstetrician in a private practice, so I went to a state-run clinic instead. I attended every lecture, discussion and class they'd offered, all while carrying a full course load. I was going to do whatever it took to get it right.

When I'd first told Brian I was pregnant, I'd also told him I didn't expect anything from him—no wedding, no support, no picket fence—he could be as involved with the baby as much or as little as he liked.

He'd responded with "You wanna get hitched?"

I'd said yes on the condition that we hold off on picking a date. I wanted to have the baby first. I thought it best to "wait and see."

His mother hadn't felt the same. Barely a week after I'd told Brian I was pregnant, she'd called from Arizona to make me an offer. She was a divorced real-estate broker who sold luxury homes in the Sonoran Desert, and her life was ruled by transactions. "I'm sending you a cheque," she'd announced. "You can use it to pay for an abortion or a wedding dress." She'd sounded so chipper and matter-of-fact, I'd thought she was joking. When the nervous chuckle I'd let out was met with silence, I'd cleared my throat and said, "Thanks."

"No problem. Just let me know what you decide. The clock's ticking."

I'd hung up the phone and gone straight to Brian. "Did you put your mother up to that?"

"No. That was all her. Welcome to the family."

When word had gotten around the music department that I was expecting, a member of the faculty had taken me aside and offered to adopt my unborn child. "You're bright and talented. You've got a promising career ahead. This could be the perfect solution for everyone." He and his wife had been unable to have a child of their own and they hadn't had much luck in dealing with the local adoption agency. He'd been my strongest advocate in the department and had helped me get my TA position, but what he was suggesting wasn't what I wanted.

"I'm keeping the baby," I'd said. "I'm sorry."

"You're sure?"

"Yes."

"When are you and Brian getting married?"

"After the baby's born, I guess."

"My advice is, don't wait. Get it done as fast as you can."

Being an unwed mother meant everyone felt entitled to tell you what to do. Tired of being badgered, I'd married Brian at the end of my first trimester in a small, simple ceremony with just our parents and a few friends from the university. It was a happy home I wanted most, not a flashy wedding. I longed for what I'd had growing up—a solid foundation, a tight-knit family, a safe haven from the noise and troubles of the world. Had my dad ever lost his temper? Sure. Was my mom ever an obstinate, emotional mess? You bet. But they were also the best example I'd ever seen of what marriage should be. This couple who'd met on a blind date and gotten married on a whim had somehow managed to keep it together for over thirty years and grow more and more in love with each other.

After we were married, Brian's mood swings became more pronounced. Whenever papers were due or exams loomed, he'd get frustrated and threaten to quit school. His anger and depression would lurch past student angst into a state of despair so deep I wasn't sure anything could bring him out of it. "I give up," would quickly turn to "I wish I was dead." I begged him to see a campus counsellor, or anyone who could offer professional help. His answer was always no, and his refusals were usually coupled with his storming out of the house or punching a wall. There were three gaping holes next to the closet in our bedroom that served as reminders of my failure to make him happy, to be a calming force, to keep trouble from our door.

Now, sitting next to my mother, I want to tell her that the reason my baby isn't coming is because the tiny, perfect being knows I've failed, and that I'm completely unprepared to be a mother.

Until this morning, I'd kept Mom at a distance, insisting I had everything under control. I'd thought that by keeping things to myself, I could solve whatever problems there were between Brian and me.

"Mom," I say, edging close to a confession.

"Yes?"

I can't do it. It's too late. "Thanks," I say.

"For what?"

"For being here."

Early the next morning, Brian drives me to the hospital. His parents are in the waiting room—his mother on one side of his dad, his dad's new wife on the other. Thankfully Brian's mom is excited enough about the baby to be cordial to the pair. My mom and dad arrive soon after, having made the two-hour drive from home with a cooler full of sandwiches and a giant Thermos of coffee for them all. When she isn't keeping everyone fed and caffeinated, Mom sneaks into the delivery room to give me support. I instantly regret that I'd listed Brian as my sole birthing coach. I'd done it in hopes that it would cause him to step up, and also to prevent Mom from seeing the truth of our situation.

Pulling one of the nurses aside, I ask her if it's too late to change my mind.

"It can cause hard feelings between family members," she says. "You don't want any additional stress on your baby's big day, do you?"

"No." The drugs are already taking effect, my contractions growing stronger.

The nurse allows Mom one last visit before drawing the line.

Unclasping the chain that bears the cross she always wears around her neck, Mom puts the cross in my hand and kisses me on the cheek. "I'd better scoot. See you and the wee one on the other side."

After several hours of crushed ice, more oxytocin, a failed vacuum extractor, and a morphine-fuelled vision where I'm surrounded by a circle of spectral grandmothers telling me to "push," the doctor finally announces, "It's a boy."

Mom drives to my house every day, after I've been released from the hospital. She washes dishes, does the laundry, cooks the meals, picks up after us.

She plays hostess to the constant flow of guests who want to meet the baby. She lends her support as I struggle to get the hang of breastfeeding. She bites her tongue as Brian's mother, who's in town for the month, constantly insists, "Let me hold that damn baby." She dries my tears when Brian's mom throws a fit and goes home early because she's not getting enough attention from Brian, or me, or her ex, or the baby. "Don't let it bother you," Mom says. "It's for the best."

A week later, when Brian is at school and all our visitors have gone, Mom gently coaxes me into taking a nap while the baby is sleeping. "I'll look after him," she says. "Go get some rest."

When I wake up, I find her sitting in a rocking chair, cradling my child. She's got him wrapped in a quilt her grandmother Tillie had made for her when she was born.

I grab my camera so I can capture the moment.

Mom looks up at me with a knowing gaze, and says, "You can come home any time you like, and stay as long as you want."

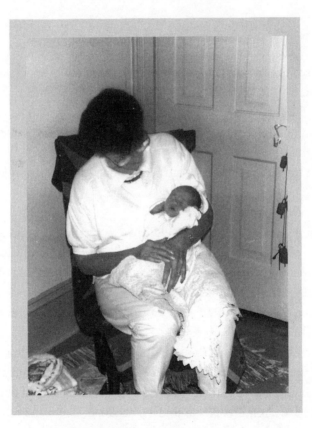

Mom holding Eldest Son, 1993

26.

It's Called Genetics

Nova Scotia, January 2018

A nurse slides a stiff canvas cuff up my arm, then gives a firm tug on its Velcro strap. "How's that feel?" she asks.

"All right."

I'm not a morning person. The sound of the Velcro sets my teeth on edge.

"It may feel a little tight at first, but that's better than it being too loose."

"Okay."

I'd gotten up at six so I could drive to the hospital and get fitted for a twenty-four-hour blood pressure monitor. My family doctor had requested I wear one since my pressure was up at my last check-up, the one in which she'd also been fairly certain she'd detected a heart murmur. All I'd wanted was an appointment for a colonoscopy. (Which I'm still waiting for.)

After walking me though the instructions, the nurse takes a sample reading before I head home. "It goes off every thirty minutes but it'll sound a warning signal first to let you know it's about to start. You'll have a few seconds to find a place to sit down and relax."

The monitor lets out an emphatic *beep* as the nurse makes a few notes on a chart. "Wow," I say. "That's loud."

"The warning signal shuts off after ten p.m., so it won't disrupt your sleep."

Thank God.

The cuff begins a slow death grip on my arm.

"Is it supposed to hurt?"

"You'll get used to it."

I shift in my seat.

"Make sure you sit still," the nurse says. "If you move too much you'll get an error. If that happens, just hang tight and the machine will reset and start again in a couple of minutes."

The first reading goes without a hitch. The nurse double-checks the monitor, which is no bigger than a deck of playing cards, then tucks it in the cloth pouch I'm supposed to wear in a sling across my chest. Handing me the chart she says, "Be sure to note the time and what you were doing before the reading *every* time it goes off."

"Is there anything I shouldn't do while I'm wearing it?"

"Other than taking a shower, no. Just do whatever you normally do. See you tomorrow before seven a.m."

"Great." I normally don't wake up until eight, so I've already thrown the test out of whack. "See you then."

TIME: 8:05 A.M.

ACTIVITY: driving

The drive home takes forty minutes. I'm still in the car when the unit beeps again with no good place to pull over. I try to keep my arm still while driving, but the machine cuts out early, registering an error. I turn onto an old logging trail and stop the car, hoping no one else will need to use the rutted dirt road while I'm there. This time the reading is a success.

TIME: 10:05, 10:35, 11:05 A.M.

ACTIVITY: vacuuming, laundry, cleaning the fridge

Since my mornings are usually spent doing chores around the house, I carry on just as the nurse advised, but I feel like I'm playing musical chairs every time the damn thing goes off. Each *beep* sets off a mad dash to find a chair, breathe deep and calm down.

TIME: 1:35, 2:05 P.M.

ACTIVITY: aspirational thinking/confronting reality

Post-lunch begins with high hopes that the day won't be a total bust. I've got plenty of writing to do—a novella to finish, incidental music to compose, the first half of a memoir to wrangle into shape—but I soon find that having my brain rattled every half hour isn't conducive to deep thinking. I'm the sort of person who needs to unplug to get anything done. No push notifications. No emails. No phone calls. No texts. No beeps.

TIME 2:25 P.M.

ACTIVITY: communing with the dead

I give up on tackling anything substantial, and sit down with my laptop to pick away at family research. Logging into the genealogy website Ancestry.com, I check to see if there are any new images posted of members of Family G. I've never stopped hoping I'll discover an old photo of Pauline.

The images I find today are mostly of tombstones—a trusty old-school resource for many genealogists. Some of my fondest childhood vacation memories are of tromping through cemeteries in Michigan with my parents, "hunting" for my kin. As I sort through the online photos, I note information and patterns I hadn't noticed in the past.

I see that in the 1930s the family began to disperse, relocating to larger towns and cities throughout Michigan and beyond. This is the farthest they've lived apart from each other in over a century.

There's a striking lack of Bible verses and religious symbols on the grave markers. Praying hands and psalms no longer accompany names and dates. By and large they've gone from being laid to rest in church-yards to being interred in public cemeteries. Had including scripture gone out of fashion? Was its absence due to a lack of funds? Or had the majority of Family G simply lost faith?

I try to imagine what it must've been like to live in a eugenics-infatuated America as a member of an "unfit family." Did the family members who left Michigan think they could escape the past by starting over someplace new? That was the path their ancestors had chosen by leaving Germany. Was that what I'd done when I'd moved to Canada? My research to this point had led me to believe that after Weller's report in 1936, certain branches of the family made a conscious effort to "forget their blood" and abandon their roots—even those who'd chosen to stay close to home.

TIME 3:05 P.M.

ACTIVITY: weighing what gets carried

I'd confirmed this deliberate "forgetting" in a series of email exchanges with a distant cousin who lives in upstate New York. Dave had first contacted me in 2002, after he'd heard the radio documentary I'd written and produced on genetic testing. Until then, neither of us had known of the other's existence. Our initial correspondence had been devoted to his questions about the testing process; I'd attempted to make it less intimidating for him. There were an ungodly number of unknowns when it came to this sort of genetic research and little if any anecdotal evidence to assuage participants' fears. We were sailing in uncharted waters. But after we'd covered those bases, we'd begun to swap stories of our ancestors, filling in gaps in each other's family trees. I'd been thrilled to find another storyteller among the branches and leaves.

Recently, I'd taken a bit of an emotional plunge by emailing Dave a few pointed questions about his family's attitudes towards cancer. I was curious as to why I'd grown up with such an intense (by some standards, morbid) awareness of the disease, while his childhood had been largely free from it. His mother, who came from my great-great-grandmother's sister's line, had been born in Ann Arbor only a few years earlier than my mom, and had died from gastric cancer in 1999. Although they were distant cousins, the two women looked remarkably alike.

"Prior to hearing my documentary, what was your understanding of cancer on your mom's side of the family?"

"Close to zero. My mother proclaimed the family history of cancer was attributable wholly to fried pork and sausage and lard and beer and the other delicacies of the German diet."

"Did people talk freely about cancer on that side of your family?" I asked.

"Hell no. It was rarely mentioned, and if broached, the questions would be quickly tabled."

"Were you aware of the family's relationship with University of Michigan Hospital? Did your family go there for medical care?"

"If there was a relationship with U of M Hospital, I never heard anything about it. I was born there but didn't set foot in there again until I was fifty-eight, when my father needed a hip replacement."

Dave's only memory of Henry Lynch's initial contact with Family G in the early 1970s was that his mother wasn't interested in participating in the research. "When Dr. Lynch came to Ann Arbor seeking blood and skin samples, my mother didn't bother." To this day, he says the attitudes of his extended family when it comes to genetic testing are "all over the map." He now realizes his mother was "scared to death of this thing. She dealt with it through her old friend, denial, and strict adherence to a healthy diet, the only thing she could control."

I can see the allure of that. Along with the threat of cancer, there's loads of emotional baggage—trunks and chests and knapsacks crammed full of grief, pain and fear. We've been carrying it with us since Johannes Haab sailed across the Atlantic in 1830, and it's any-one's guess how long before that. Some days I wish I could forget what I know, scrap the screenings and the latest research and the whole previvor thing. If not for my mother's sense of duty echoing in my heart and the profound strength of her love, I don't know where I'd be. Maybe that's the murmur the doctor was hearing.

TIME: 4:05, 4:35 P.M.
ACTIVITY: walking the dog/clearing my head
I walk the dog down a dirt road to a narrow lane that leads to the sea. The wind is raw and the sun is setting. I need to be by the water's edge as the day's light wanes. A place where one thing ends and another begins.

TIME: 9:05 P.M.

ACTIVITY: watching TV/contemplating fate

I put the leftovers from supper away and fold the laundry, then wander upstairs to catch the news. All the 24/7 networks—CNN, MSNBC, Fox and even the CBC—are repeatedly running excerpts from a press conference that had taken place earlier in the day in which the White House physician, Dr. Ronny Jackson, had declared that President Trump was "in excellent health."

When asked how Trump can be so healthy, despite his lack of exercise and love of fast food, Dr. Jackson had said, "It's called genetics. He has incredibly good genes, and it's just the way God made him."

Bully for him.

One commentator points out Trump himself has regularly touted the superiority of his genes. For instance:

"I always said winning is somewhat, maybe innate. Maybe it's something you have, you know, you have the *winning* gene."

"I have great genes and all that stuff which, I'm a believer in."

"I have a certain gene. I'm a gene believer."

"Do we believe the gene thing? I mean I do."

"I consider my health, stamina and strength one of my greatest assets. The world has watched me for many years and can so testify—great genes!"

"You have to have the right genes."

The president's glowing bill of health comes hard on the heels of yet another report of Trump voicing contentious views on immigration.

"Why are we having all these people from shithole countries come here?"

"Why do we need more Haitians?"

Supposedly, he'd rather have more migrants from Norway.

This from a man who mocks the disabled, calls Mexicans "rapists" and who stated:

"All men are created equal. Well, it's not true."

Between a slew of commercials for diet programs and gym memberships, an ad from a well-known DNA testing service runs, featuring the rugged but friendly voice of a man who asks me to imagine, "You

can have any car you want, but it will be the only car you'll ever have."
As he goes on about how well I'd need to take care of said car, scenes
of childhood flash on the screen—a boy riding a bike, kids jumping in
a swimming hole, teens sitting around a campfire. As a young man
takes a stroll with his sweetheart, the guy changes his tune and says,
"Well, you know you're not going to get only one car in your lifetime,
but you *are* only going to get one body, and only one mind, and that
body and mind feels terrific right now, but it has to last you a lifetime.
This year, learn more about your body. Understand your DNA."

TIME: 10:05 P.M.
ACTIVITY: failing to fall asleep
What exactly are "great" genes?

The phrase gets breezily tossed off in everyday conversation—as
a compliment, as justification for success, as a boast of superiority.
"Bad" genes get blamed for our shortcomings—physical, professional,
academic. It all feels grossly ignorant and sinister.

Science has given the human race the ability to decipher our
DNA, but can we be trusted to take proper care of it?

Mrs. Matilda A. Wheeler died Wednesday evening at
her home, 203 N. Lewis Street, after a brief illness. She
was born June 23, 1876 in Freedom Township, the daughter
of J. Frederick Gross and Katherine Haab Gross.
Mrs. Wheeler married Oscar Wheeler, October 4, 1900.
He preceded her in death in 1945.

—from the *Saline Observer*, December 20, 1951

27.

When Sally Met Larry

Michigan State College, December 28, 1951
Tillie's granddaughter Sarah Anne stares into a full-length mirror
hanging on the back of the door to her dorm room in Williams Hall.
Leaning forward she deftly applies her lipstick, then pinches a piece
of folded tissue between her lips to set it.

Her roommate, Ibby, lets out a long whistle. "You look great, Sal."

Sarah Anne has been "Sally" for years, but Ibby insists her best
friend is better served by the punch of a single syllable.

Sally takes a drag on a cigarette the two girls have been sharing.
"You really think I look all right?"

"That sailor boy won't know what hit him."

The two co-eds had returned to campus from the holidays early.
Sally had planned to tuck in at the library for the duration, thinking
that solitude and a few good books would be the best remedy for
her grief. Her grandmother's death, two weeks before Christmas,
had struck her as incredibly unfair: Gram Tillie had loved the

holidays. She was also feeling bereft that she hadn't had a chance to say goodbye.

Ibby had insisted a night on the town might be the better medicine. To that end, she'd arranged a blind date for Sally with a childhood friend of her current beau, a young sailor named Larry who was home on holiday leave. "I predict that by night's end he'll be down on bended knee."

"Don't get ahead of yourself, Ibby. I only agreed to one date."

"Sometimes one is all it takes."

Sally had gone home to her parents' house after the funeral, and had wound up regretting it. While her younger brother and sister, now thirteen and six, had grown like weeds, her parents seemed to have aged a thousand years. Her father had been in and out of the hospital for chronic emphysema and a bad back, leaving him more out of work than in it. Her mother, trying to make up for what they lacked, was tired and overworked and always anticipating the worst. Tillie's death had heightened all of Alice's fears and insecurities, which she never kept to herself. "What will happen when I get sick?" "I'm not getting any younger, you know." "How will I survive it?" "How will we get by?"

"You'll manage, Mom." Sally had said, again and again. "Just like Gram did. We'll cross that bridge when we come to it."

This sort of talk was all she'd had left in her, and likely all that Alice could handle.

The two of them had gone round and round before she'd left for her first year at university in August—with Alice taking every opportunity to point out how much work she'd have to do by herself with Sally gone, and Sally wishing out loud that her mother could say she was proud of her just once. She'd earned every penny she'd needed for tuition, board and books, but all Alice could do was remind her, "Watch your pocketbook. We won't be able to help if you get in a pinch."

While other mothers had sent her classmates loving cards and care packages, Alice had sent letters of complaint.

I've been trying to figure out how we can get along better. I know I'm at fault in a lot of ways, but I don't seem to know how to go about helping it. Maybe when you come home we can sit down together and air our grievances.

There'd been no "how are your classes going?" or even a "love, Mom."

I managed to get the dishes done last night—so there's not too many this morning. Now I'm going to do what's left (yes, really). Keep your fingers crossed we sell all the pups this weekend. Daddy and Jamie need new shoes. By fall, with any luck at all, we should be better off financially than we have been, and also have the place in better shape.
    Toodle-doo
    Mom.

For as long as Sally could remember, headaches, exhaustion and long bouts of reminiscing about "the good old days" had hindered her mother from doing household chores. She'd learned early on how to do whatever needed doing in order to keep herself and their home presentable. She'd done it in hopes that her mother might reward her for her efforts with a bit of affection. All she'd gotten was a heap of guilt—and even more on this last visit. "Can't you stay a little longer? There's a mountain of laundry to be done and I'm sure your daddy would love you to cook for him," her mother had said. Even her sister had bitterly complained at her going: "I don't see why *she* always has to go away."

Sally couldn't see why her mother had to pick at every wrong, hurt, loss or illness so they'd never heal or go away. She refused to live like that. She was determined to go forward in the direction of her dreams.

"Wait," Sally says, stopping Ibby on the stairs down to the dormitory lobby. "Are you sure I look all right?"

"Stop fretting," Ibby says. "You're perfect." Peeking into the lobby, she adds, "Chin up, he's here."

Standing beside the fireplace is a young man who, with his blue eyes, wavy brown hair and skinny build, bears a striking resemblance to Frank Sinatra in *On the Town*. Sally wonders if he likes to sing.

"Larry," Ibby says. "This is Sal." She gives Sally a wink, then sneaks away.

The pair exchange greetings then make their way out of the building, passing beneath a wide Tudor arch inscribed with the words *Every day in thy life is a leaf in thy history*. The street lamps that line the walkway cast golden moons on the snow-covered lawn.

That first date turns into two, then three, then four, and by the end of a painfully short week, a twenty-year-old sailor named Larry will have given eighteen-year-old Sally the two most valuable things he possesses: his class ring from Owosso High, and his heart.

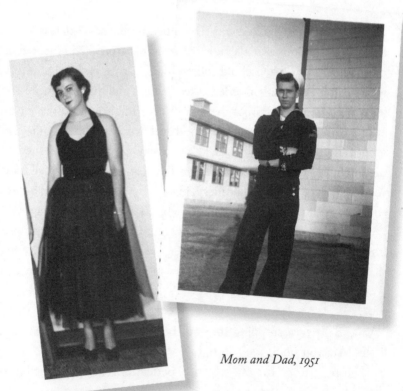

Mom and Dad, 1951

January 10, 1952, Michigan State College

Larry—You mentioned in your letter that perhaps I wouldn't believe what you had told me. Well I do believe you. I guess I am a rather strange person, but I believe people until they have proven to me that they aren't worthy of my belief and if that time comes, in my estimation, they aren't worth trying to believe anymore.

Honestly, I believe things have happened to me since I met you. If I didn't think a lot of you, I wouldn't be wearing your ring right now. It gives me a very proud and happy feeling to know that you wanted me to wear it and I do so with pride and affection.

I will send you a picture this afternoon. Please don't forget that you said you would send me one of you.

Love Sally

January 15, 1952, Naval Air Station Memphis

Dear Sally,

Guess What? I'm the happiest guy in the US Navy! Today I received a letter and a picture of the most wonderful girl I know, honest.

You haven't been out of my mind since I've come back. I sure wish I wasn't far away. I would like to take you out every nite and even more if you would let me, but if you will give me a chance someday I'll make up for lost time.

Thanks for the picture, it's really swell. I've got it in my locker, so when I open the door, there you are.

Love, Larry

PS I hope with all my heart I'll never give you a reason to disbelieve me.

January 16, 1952 Michigan State College

Dear Larry,

This is the second letter I've started to you this week. I was feeling lonesome in the first one and wishing you were here, and especially thinking of the week before at the same time. I decided

that it was better, in the mood I was in, not to finish it, for I would
be saying things I should save until we see each other again.

Larry: please don't think that you ever have anything to make
up to me. I wish, just as much as you do that you were here and
we could see more of each other. Perhaps this waiting time will
mean that we will be closer than if we had been together.

All my love,
Sal

January 18, 1952, Naval Air Station Memphis
You know I've read your letter five or six times today? Sally, you've
done something to me, and I like it very much.

I wish I could write and tell you how much you mean to me.
I've tried, but I get all mixed up. I guess I could tell you better
than I can put it on paper.

Remember I'll be thinking of you (as if I could ever forget you).
Write soon,
Love always,
Larry

January 21, 1952 Michigan State College
Dear Larry,

I think the things we have to tell each other are about the
same.

You said that you would be thinking of me "as if you could
ever forget me." That expresses my feelings exactly—I can't forget
you, and every night and day I think of how wonderful it would
be if you were here. Please know that I'm willing to wait however
long it takes. As long as you are in my heart I am happy.

All my love,
Sally

January 24, 1952, Naval Air Station Memphis
You know Sal, there's a part in your last letter on which I'm going
to base my future hopes. It's the part where you said you would be

"willing to wait" for me. I believe you Sally. Do you know why
I believe you? It's because I've fallen in love with you. I couldn't
wait any longer to tell you, and I hope you have guessed it by now.
If I don't get leave after this, it might be a long time before I get
home and I sure want you to know how much you mean to me.

All my love,

Larry

January 28, 1952 Michigan State College
Larry,

I love you too, very much, and as far as waiting goes, I'll wait
forever and two days after forever has come if need be for you.
Naturally I miss you very much and want to be near you, but
I realize that our love for each other is the important thing and as
long as we have that, everything else is minor.

You may start planning or hoping for the future as of now, for
as far as I'm concerned you will be in my hopes, plans, prayers and
dreams until we are together to fulfill them.

It seems rather wonderful and strange to be saying those
things to someone whom I thought I didn't know at all, but every
day I find I am closer to you. Do you realize we have known each
other for a month now? You couldn't mean any more to me had
I known you for years.

Goodnight Larry, I'll see you in my dreams.

All my love,

Sally

February 1, 1952, Naval Air Station Memphis
Hello Angel,

I received your letter today and every time I read it I get a
wonderful warm feeling. This is what I've wanted all my life and
I know you're the only one who ever has, does, or ever will make
me feel the way I do now.

Do you remember in your letter you mentioned we have
known each other for a month? The element of time is a funny

thing. To me you're a girl I've had in my mind for a long long time, so we're really old friends, but now that I've met you, flesh and blood, you're more than a friend, you're the woman I love.

All my love,

Larry

February 4, 1952, Michigan State College
My Darling Larry,

Your letter came this morning and since then I've read it about twenty times. It seems so wonderful to know that we feel the same about each other. It's really clear our love is here to stay, not for a year but ever and a day. You said it was too bad your dreams can't come true. Together we can make our dreams come true no matter what they are.

You mean all the world to me.

From, "the woman you love," Sally

February 15, 1952, Naval Air Station Memphis
Dear Sal,

Did you ever hear of a place called Atsugi? That's where I'll be stationed. It's about 40 miles out of Tokyo and that's all I know about it, except it's a naval station.

I also know I love you, that's for darn sure.

Larry

Except for a short leave where Larry says goodbye to his family and meets Sally's parents, they will be apart for the next two and a half years.

One week after his return from Atsugi, in the summer of 1954, they marry.

28.

At Least It Wasn't Cancer

Terre Haute, Indiana, October 1993

The phone rings and I jump to answer it before it can ring again. I'd been up all night nursing my baby through his first cold. It's nearly noon, and he's finally fallen asleep.

"Hello?" I say in a half-whisper.

"Hey, kiddo."

"Hey, Dad."

"Got a minute?"

"Sure."

"I'm calling to let you know that Alice passed away this morning."

I let his words sink in. "Oh, Dad. I don't know what to say."

"You don't have to say anything. I just thought you'd want to know right away."

My eyes fill with tears. "Thanks."

"I can call back later if you like."

"No. It's okay. I just need a second."

"Take your time."

I can't remember a time when I hadn't been expecting to hear that my grandmother had died. She was perpetually planning her exit, taking last bows, saying goodbye. Now that the moment has arrived, I'm a pathetic mess of hormones, sadness and regret. I can feel my breast milk letting down, my T-shirt going damp, as salty tears stream down my face. "Was it peaceful?" I ask. It's the first thing that comes to mind.

"Yes," Dad says, "she was in her bed at the nursing home when it happened. Her heart finally gave up the ghost."

Alice's voice whispers in my head. *At least it wasn't cancer.*

Strange as it seems, I can't believe she's gone. "I just saw her two weeks ago and she seemed fine." (Or at least as fine as any eighty-seven-year-old with a pacemaker and an extremely short colon.)

"At least she got to meet her newest great-grandchild before she went."

"I should've gone to visit her sooner."

"Don't beat yourself up over it. You did the best you could."

"I should've guessed it would be our last time together. She kept saying how ready she was to die, and that she figured the reason she wasn't dead yet was because God didn't want her."

Dad sighs. "And what did you say to that?"

"I told her that God just needed to find something for her to do, to keep her out of trouble."

"Well, I guess he finally figured it out."

"How's Mom?" I ask, taking a tearful breath.

"She's doing all right. She's a tough one, my Sal."

"Anything I can do for her?"

"Come home when you can."

"I'm on my way."

I pack some clothes in a suitcase and fill the baby's diaper bag with what we'll need for the next few days. There's no time to track down Brian, so I leave a note on the kitchen table. He's in the last year of his undergrad, so it doesn't make sense for him to drop everything and make the trip. I'm not sure I want him to come, anyway.

The first few weeks after the baby's birth had been difficult. I was perpetually sleep-deprived, and Brian's academic schedule was filled with courses he'd either dropped in the past or had put off taking until now, which he needed to complete to graduate. This had made for a perfect storm of weariness and frustration.

One night, when Brian had been in a rehearsal, a mutual friend had stopped by the house to say he was worried about his state of mind. "He's been doing that thing where he says he wants to quit."

Brian had been saying the same thing to me since the start of the semester, but whenever I'd offered to help, he'd gotten angry and shut me down. "He always talks like that. You know how he gets."

"He also said he's nothing but a big fuck-up and that he doesn't want to live."

"Was he drunk?"

"Yeah."

Drinking always made it worse.

Brian had been spending a lot of time away from the house, studying, practicing, blowing off steam with friends. I'd thought it was because he'd needed some time to ease into being a dad. "Do you think he was serious or just talking shit?"

"I don't know. It scared me. That's why I'm here. When I asked him if he was going to be okay, he changed the subject and started talking about auditioning for one of the army bands. He thinks if he gets in, his problems will disappear because all he'll have to do is play."

I wasn't too keen on my baby's father enlisting in the army, even as a musician. I was also hurt that Brian hadn't mentioned any of this to me.

"Thanks for letting me know. I'll try talking to him about it tonight."

"Keep me posted, okay?"

"All right."

I tried talking to Brian, but our talk had turned into yet another fight. "Why can't you leave me the fuck alone?" he'd yelled. "You're driving me crazy!" After that, he'd taken a set of golf clubs his father had given him for his birthday and proceeded to snap each of the irons in half across his knee. Since then, he'd been sleeping on the couch. He hadn't asked to come back to our bed and I hadn't issued an invitation. I'd told myself it was fine for now, since the baby wasn't yet sleeping through the night. We'd work things out—or I'd find a way out—eventually.

❧

As sad as I am over Alice's passing, it's a relief to be at my parents' house, thinking of something else besides my crumbling marriage.

The baby, despite his cold, puts on gurgles and smiles for everyone. The biggest grins, of course, go to my mom. It's a joy to watch them together. Mom recites nursery rhymes ("This little piggy went to market"), even her recipe for hollandaise sauce ("don't forget the nutmeg"), as he stares at her with wide, adoring eyes.

The morning of Alice's memorial service is cold and overcast. I ride along with my parents so Mom can have more time with the baby. Dad drives on the back roads to the funeral home as turning leaves, fields of ripe pumpkins and soybeans set for harvest blur past the windows in a river of fiery hues under the slate grey sky.

The service is exactly as expected. Alice's children, grandchildren, and a handful of friends and acquaintances gather in the generic-looking chapel to pay their last respects. The flower arrangements boast the same kinds of blossoms as had graced the church on her "official" wedding day—zinnias, marigolds, dahlias. The organist plays tasteful arrangements of Alice's favourite hymns, and the preacher from my aunt's church delivers scripture readings, prayers and a short sermon. One of the nurses from the rest home fondly recalls Alice as "a lover of basketball, a wonderful storyteller, and an attentive listener." Citing Alice's training as a teacher and a social worker, she says, "She was helpful to everyone around her to the very end. She was a true woman of God who always cared for others. She was a compassionate friend."

On our way home, we stop at a roadside diner for coffee. After changing the baby's diaper, I sit and nurse him in the back of the car until he falls asleep. As I tuck him into his car seat, Dad comes out of the diner and motions for me to roll down the window. "Can you check on Mom?" he asks. "She's been in the ladies' room for a while now."

"Sure."

The ladies' room consists of two sinks, a hand-towel roller with a pitted mirror and three toilet stalls with metal doors. I can't see Mom, but the door to the last stall is shut and I can hear crying.

"Mom?" I say, bending over and looking under it. I spot the pair of black patent pumps she'd bought at JC Penney when I was in high school. "Are you okay?"

I hear her blow her nose and fumble with the latch on the door. "Come on in," she says.

I slip into the narrow stall and close the door behind me. She's standing to one side of the toilet with her back against a wall of drab beige tiles. Her blouse is half tucked in her skirt and her makeup is mostly rubbed off. A swipe of blush at the edge of each temple is all that remains.

I tug a length of toilet paper from the roll and hand it to her. "Dad's worried about you. Are you all right?"

She shakes her head and starts crying again.

I stare at the bright blue water in the toilet bowl. The air is thick with the chemical scent of truck stops and hospitals. *As if anything could make our shit not stink.* I reach for Mom's hand.

Shoulders quaking, she says, "I don't know who that woman was talking about today."

"What do you mean?"

"When that nurse stood up at the service and started saying all those nice things about Alice, all I could think was that she couldn't be talking about *my* mother."

"Oh, Mom," I say, wrapping my arms around her. "I'm so sorry."

"Why couldn't she ever be that person with me?"

I knew the Alice the nurse had described. She had showered me with attention, passed on her deep love for history and the written word, and talked with me openly and honestly about cancer. She'd trusted me with her stories.

The last time I'd seen her, she'd told me she'd made arrangements to donate her body to science. "So I can go on helping others."

But she had never been able to show that same generosity of heart to my mother.

Knowing that she was still longing for Alice's love was almost more than I could bear. I want to tell her that she's the kind of mother I want to be, the woman I hope to become, but the only words I can find are, "I love you, Mom."

☙

In early December, two months after Alice's death, the following headline appears on the front page of the *New York Times*.

SCIENTISTS ISOLATE GENE THAT CAUSES
CANCER OF COLON

SCREENING TEST FORECAST

CRUCIAL EARLY WARNING MAY BE POSSIBLE FOR
FAMILIES WITH HISTORY OF THE DISEASE

This must've been what Dr. Lynch had been hinting at when he'd told my mother they were getting closer to cracking the code on the family's cancer. No wonder she'd willingly signed over her blood and tissue samples to Henry after her surgery.

According to the article, researchers looking for ways in which cancer begins in the body discovered that a flaw in an individual's DNA could cause a certain type of colorectal cancer. More precisely, when the MSH2 gene, responsible for activating a protein essential to our cells' repair of damaged DNA, is defective, its ability to function as a genetic caretaker is at risk. In some instances, other genes share the load in this kind of repair signalling, but for some tissues in the body, there is no backup for the job that MSH2 does. Much like the spellcheck function in a word processing program, MSH2 serves to alert the cells' repair function to correct mistakes. With the "spell-check" gone, errors accumulate and the result is cancer—of the colon, uterus, small intestine, pancreas, ovaries and kidney—the exact kinds of cancers Family G has suffered from for generations.

Now that a link between this specific gene and certain cancers has been made, the next steps include verifying a pattern of inheritance within families where those cancers are prevalent and developing a test that can detect the defective gene. Those testing positive can undergo colonoscopies and other screenings to discover cancer at its earliest stages. Those who test negative can rest easy knowing they're free from this particular threat.

As Dr. Bert Vogelstein, a lead author on a report announcing the isolation of the gene, explains: "The great thing about the diagnostic implications of this work is that deaths are entirely preventable. If you know you have a mutation in this gene, you can take steps to keep yourself from dying."

Mom could finally have the proof she's always wanted "to make doctors sit up and listen." And evidently, so might a lot of other people too. According to the article, "as many as 1 in 200 people, or more than a million Americans, are thought to carry the mutation, most of them without any knowledge of their inherent risk."

As promising as the discovery sounds, it's not a thornless rose. The scientists interviewed for the article estimate that the test, once developed, will cost $1,000 per person. Those who test positive for the gene may well find their insurance premiums skyrocket or be dropped by their provider altogether. A genetic test for hereditary predisposition to cancer is something for which the industry has no standard. (The breast cancer genes for BRCA1 and 2 will not be discovered until 1994 and '95, respectively.) Furthermore, women who carry the MSH2 gene have the additional burden of being at significantly higher risk for uterine and ovarian cancer. Dr. Francis Collins of the National Center for Human Genome Research expressed his concern to the *Times*, "It raises the possibility that one might consider prophylactic surgery, that is, removal of the ovaries. Researchers do not yet know whether or at what age such a step might be advised. Women may find themselves in a fearful tussle between the desire to have children, and the concern that if they wait just a bit too long, they will develop cancer."

Is this what my family has?

Is it already lurking inside me?

Do I want to know the answer?

29.

What Do I Do?

Scots Bay, Nova Scotia, April 2018

Once a week I visit an online forum devoted to Lynch syndrome. It's populated by people of various ages from around the world, each of us at a different stage in coping with the condition. Many participants are working through their first, second or even third cancers, their minds occupied by surgeries, aftercare and treatment. The majority of them weren't tested for Lynch syndrome until after they'd been diagnosed with cancer.

A few, like me, are previvors—people who tested positive for Lynch syndrome without having had cancer. Many are in their late twenties or early thirties. Most have only recently received their results. I'm the seasoned veteran in the group. Newbies often ask for a roll call: Where is everyone from? How long have you known you've had Lynch syndrome? How old were you at your first cancer diagnosis? What kind of cancer was it? What surgeries have you had? If you're a previvor, how long have you known? How old are you now? What's your mutation? (There are now five different gene mutations associated with Lynch syndrome: MLH1, MSH2, MSH6, PMS2 and EPCAM. MSH2 was the first.)

Nova Scotia, Canada. Previvor since 2002. Prophylactic
hysterectomy at 45. I'm now 49. Mutation: MSH2

Topics of our conversations include: colonoscopy tips, chemotherapy woes, insurance coverage, drug trials, scientific studies, post-op diet, and the pros and cons of prophylactic hysterectomy. We make fart jokes, poo puns and teasingly argue over who has the hardest colonoscopy prep. We also support one another through the worst aspects of the disease—from cancer diagnoses to family deaths to finding out one of our children has tested positive for Lynch.

We hold each other's hands across cyberspace as we wait for test results, doctors' appointments, and surgeries. Everyone agrees, waiting sucks.

One month since my Lynch diagnosis and I'm still trying to get my baseline screenings. I'm a colon cancer survivor and insurance doesn't want to cover me. What do I do?

Has anyone been diagnosed with Lynch before having children? How did you come to the decision to have or to forgo having children?

Getting ready to have a hysterectomy at 35. I've heard horror stories about it. Obviously it beats getting cancer, but how bad is it?

My surgeon insisted I should have a surgery to remove my colon as well as total hysterectomy and mastectomy. Any thoughts?

Anyone here had their entire right liverlobe removed?

I am extremely concerned about my kids. I want to have them tested as soon as possible.

I have yet to fully understand this mutation and its implications. Does being positive with Lynch syndrome mean I will definitely get cancer? I feel like I've been handed a death warrant.

I'm a 10 year ovarian cancer survivor (caught at age 44). My sister has had four different cancers over the last 40 or so years, and our dad passed away after his third round of colon cancer at age 79.

His mother and brothers also had colon cancer. I have two sons,
and both of them will be doing the testing in the near future.
Hopefully they'll be lucky and it won't have passed on to them.

Waiting for results is horribly anxiety producing. I know whatever
will be, will be, but my brain is trying to convince me I'm dying.
I hate this.

One post from a regular member of the group catches my attention:

I recently used a private lab service to get my daughter tested.
They specialize in hereditary cancer genes, so it was thorough and
fast. Would highly recommend.

I think back to just after Christmas, when Eldest Son had submitted his paperwork to the provincial health care system so he could enter the queue for genetic testing. I'd tried to be positive when he'd said it could take up to a year to be called for an appointment, but for the past three months, I've been worrying about what that wait could mean.

Cruising the private lab's website, I click on and watch an information video, then call one of their lab techs to ask questions.

"Your test analyzes thirty genes, including BRCA1 and BRCA2. Does it also include the genes for Lynch syndrome?"

"Yes."

"*All* of them?"

"Yes."

"Including MSH2?" I need to be sure.

"Yes."

The lab tech cheerfully adds, "Genetic counselling is also included in the price of the test package."

For a few hundred dollars and Eldest Son's complete medical history, they'll provide a spit kit and all the information he needs to take the test. "Patients get their results in about four weeks."

The medical system in Nova Scotia has never let me down, so the thought of skirting around it makes me uneasy. Still, the sooner my son gets the test done, the sooner he'll know what his next steps should be. If he's negative, he'll have one less thing to tackle in life. If he's positive, he'll need to get the ball rolling for annual tests and screenings. (And I'll have to find a way to deal with the guilt.)

As I weigh the option in my mind, I think of how overjoyed my mother had been when Dr. Lynch had informed her that a test to determine if her children carried the mutation was finally available. "We did it!" she'd proudly proclaimed. "No more wondering. No more begging for colonoscopies. No more doctors saying: 'it's in your head,' or 'adhesions,' or 'just the flu.'" It'd taken far longer than anyone had expected to get to that point—seven years from the time Mom had signed the pink release forms to donate her tumour samples to Dr. Lynch, to when the test was ready.

In my mind, the discovery of the Family G mutation is the stuff of legend, with Mom's DNA serving as the key to the breakthrough. Without Mom, there would be no test.

Now, I find myself wondering what those years had been like for the researchers in the lab where the discovery had been made. Not long after Henry had obtained Mom's samples in the early '90s, they'd been sent to a lab at Johns Hopkins headed up by Dr. Bert Vogelstein— the same man who'd first discovered the link between MSH2 and cancer. He was also the man who'd gone on to isolate all the causative genes for Lynch syndrome.

I've reached out to Dr. Lynch several times over the past few years—first to invite him to participate in my radio documentary about genetic testing, and then more recently to follow up on a few questions I had about the history of Lynch syndrome. He always answers my emails within a few hours of my sending them. He's just turned ninety, but still comes into the lab every day. He's been a part of my life for so long, I don't think twice anymore about contacting him. Dr. Vogelstein is a different story. He's currently the director of the Ludwig Center for Cancer Research at Johns Hopkins and his papers have been cited over 300,000 times. According to Wikipedia, that's "more often than those of any other scientist, in any discipline, in recorded history."

I have no idea if Bert Vogelstein will respond if I send him an email, but it's worth a try.

Besides, I need to do something to clear my head as I work up the courage to call my son. On the one hand, I don't want him to feel as if I'm rushing him to get tested. On the other, I need him to know I'll do whatever it takes to help him get it done.

> Dear Dr. Vogelstein,
>
> I am Ami McKay, a published author, and proud member of Aldred Warthin's 'Family G' as first mentioned in medical literature in 1913.
>
> I'm currently writing a genetic memoir, based on my family's history in regards to medical research relating to Lynch syndrome, and my personal experiences as an unaffected carrier who has lived with a Lynch syndrome diagnosis for nearly twenty years. The book spans from 1895 when my great-great-aunt Pauline, "the seamstress," first told Warthin of the family's history of cancer to the present.
>
> In recent correspondence with Dr. Henry Lynch, I discussed his collaboration with you during the exciting period of time when the causative mutation for MSH2 was discovered, as well as the subsequent development of a genetic test that would identify carriers of the gene in my family.
>
> The early '90s were an intense time for me as well, as my mother was diagnosed with colon cancer and I was pregnant with my first child. My mother had developed a friendly relationship with Dr. Lynch during his years of researching our family and was more than happy to donate tissue and blood samples to "help the cause." It's my understanding that with Henry's encouragement, they found their way to your lab. Sadly, my mom passed away in 2007 due to complications from a second CRC, but her open nature and her commitment to spreading the word about Lynch syndrome lives on and has served as the inspiration behind many of her kin choosing to undergo genetic testing, including myself. (I was tested in 2001.)

As I wrap up my research for the book, I'm hoping that you might answer a few questions I have about your work on the MSH2 connection to Lynch syndrome and the development of the genetic test. Thanks in advance for any insights you can give.

After asking a series of detailed questions about his research, I close by posing a more personal query.

This may seem like a funny question, but I'm wondering if you listen to music when you work in your office or in the lab? Is there any music that sticks out for you from that time period or in general? (Although I'm a full-time writer, my graduate studies were in musicology, so I'm always interested in the intersection between music and science, even on a personal level.)

I obsessively reread the email several times before pressing *send*.

I'm not sure why I'm so nervous about reaching out to him. My mother had been adamant during my upbringing that I not fear doctors. "They're human, just like you or me or anybody else." That of course meant that they, too, could be wrong. Mom had set an excellent example for my siblings and me by always looking doctors straight in the eye, keeping a small notepad handy to record their comments, and holding firm to her belief that everyone is entitled to a second opinion. "Never assume that one person knows everything about anything."

I've had to do my share of educating medical professionals when it comes to Lynch syndrome. Even now it's not as widely known among general practitioners as it should be. My intent, of course, isn't to be a Lynch-splainer, but rather to make sure nothing falls through the cracks. Lynch syndrome cancers are swift and aggressive. Failure to get screened in a timely fashion could be fatal. I'm not averse to whipping out an accordion file full of medical records to make my case.

Taking a deep breath, I finally pick up my phone and call Eldest Son.

"Hey, you."

"Hey, Mom."

"Got a minute to talk?"

"Sure."

I tell him about the private lab and that I'll gladly pay for his test. "I'll send you a link to their website. Once you've looked it over, let me know what you think."

"I'll do it," he says without hesitation.

"Are you sure?"

"Yes. I don't want to wait."

Just as our conversation ends, my phone dings. Dr. Vogelstein has sent a reply.

> Hi Ami—
>
> One question is easy to answer: I'm listening to "Sing, Sing, Sing" right now.
>
> The others will take a bit of time. Are you in a rush? The next two months are incredibly hectic for me. After that, we could chat.
>
> B

We're going to get along just fine.

30.

When Sally Met Henry

Ann Arbor, Michigan, 1965

In the fall of 1965, two medical researchers from Nebraska arrive at the University of Michigan at the invitation of Dr. A.J. French, head of the Department of Pathology. French had recently read a paper written by one member of the team, Dr. Henry Lynch, a thirty-seven-year-old medical oncologist with an extensive background in genetics. Lynch's detailed account of a family with a seemingly strong predilection for cancer had reminded French of Family G and the studies that'd been carried out by his predecessors, Aldred Warthin and Carl Weller.

Weller had died suddenly in 1956, and in the aftermath, research on Family G had come to an abrupt halt. The department's records and accompanying pathologic materials pertaining to the family had been archived in a small closet within the offices of the Department of Human Genetics. Lynch and his colleague, Anne Krush, a social worker specializing in medical research, hope that a close examination of the Family G material will provide insight into their current work: a continuing study of a family in Nebraska who show a strong tendency towards certain cancers. The medical histories of that family had been limited in scope, but what data they had been able to collect had led the pair to strongly suspect that the family's woes were being caused by something they'd named "cancer family syndrome." Problem was, observations based on such a small study had only gotten them so far. The prospect of poring over seventy-five years' worth of data and pathologic documentation of Family G excites the pair to no end. They're hoping it will provide a path to proving their hunch.

And, after examining every file, slide and report in the Family G archive, the pair is more convinced than ever of their thesis. While Family G isn't connected to the Nebraska family by blood, Lynch quickly sees striking similarities between them, specifically in the way certain cancers have presented across generations.

Anne Krush writes down the names of the youngest members of Family G at the time of Weller's death. "We should see if any of them still live in the area."

"I should warn you," Dr. French says before sending them on their way, "there were some turn-offs among family members the last time they were approached."

Over the course of the next few years, Lynch and Krush search out as many living members of Family G as they can—gathering medical reports and conducting interviews with both family members and their physicians along the way. Whether it's Krush's unshakable enthusiasm or Lynch's dogged belief in what they're pursuing, the two are greeted, for the most part, with cooperation and good will. One relative leads to another, and then another, and then another, and soon Lynch and Krush find themselves travelling beyond the confines of Ann Arbor.

Henry Lynch drives to nearby Ypsilanti to meet with Otto and Oscar Haab, a pair of brothers who own a local diner. The three men trade stories over bratwurst and beers—the Haab boys telling tales of their family exploits, and Lynch, in turn, regaling them with memories of his time as a sixteen-year-old gunner during WWII and his brief stint as a boxer under the ring name Hammerin' Hank. By the time Lynch says goodbye, he has been declared an honorary member of Family G.

In 1969, Anne Krush ambitiously spearheads a trip to Germany to track down any family members who might remain in the rural village Johannes Haab left behind in 1830. Together with Lynch and his wife, June, a nurse, she travels to Plattenhardt to meet a Lutheran minister who puts them in touch with the remaining relatives who still live in the area. Through a mix of broken German and English, more connections are made, more insights gained.

Upon their return, the team makes contact with Matilda Gross Wheeler's daughters. Now in their fifties and sixties, they are scattered geographically but still in close touch with each other. The sisters admire Anne's thoughtful approach and Henry's forthright nature. Being able to speak openly with the knowledgeable pair about the disease comes as a great relief, especially as they recently lost their youngest brother, Bud, to pancreatic cancer at forty-nine.

Doris, who lives in South Bend, Indiana, had endometrial cancer at forty-three.

Alice, who lives farther south in Indianapolis, has just recently recovered from colorectal cancer, as has her son, Jamie, who was only twenty-six at the time of his diagnosis. Alice is so impressed by Lynch and Krush that she immediately puts them in contact with the gastroenterologist who'd overseen both her and her son's care at the Indiana University School of Medicine.

Alice's eldest daughter, Sally, agrees to speak with the team, but has many questions.

"What exactly are you looking for?"

"What do you plan to do with my information?"

"Why do you need to know about my children?"

She's happily married to the love of her life and living in a comfy little house in rural Indiana. Their four healthy children keep them on their toes—two boys in their early teens and two little girls. The youngest—me—has just learned to walk. Sally will do anything to protect them.

The researchers tell her, "You can give us as much or as little information as you like, but the more we learn about you and your family, the better understanding we'll have of what your risks are and how to help you."

Filling out the team's forms and questionnaires, she thinks of her children, so young and full of promise. *I hope to God they'll never have to think about any of this.*

In April of 1970, Henry Lynch attends the annual meeting of the American College of Physicians in Philadelphia to present the team's most recent findings on Family G. To date, his ideas on hereditary cancer syndromes have fallen on deaf ears. Most members of the medical research community continue to reject the notion that any cancer could be caused by inherited factors. After meeting with members of Family G, Lynch is convinced that some are. The data he's collected in the past few years has helped him form what he feels to be the cardinal principles of "cancer family syndrome":

1. Increased occurrences of site-specific cancers.

2. Increased incidence of multiple primary cancers.

3. Evidence of autosomal dominant inheritance patterns. (The disorder need only be present in one parent to be passed on.)

4. Early age onset of cancer.

These four observations will become the guideposts for hereditary cancer research into the twenty-first century.

Before he ends his talk, Lynch acknowledges the work that came before he and Anne Krush arrived on the scene. He says, "We are indeed fortunate to have available to us a larger cancer-prone kindred in whom meticulous pathologic verification of tumours has been attained through several generations during the past seventy-five years. In addition, the many years devoted to investigations of this kindred have resulted in an unusually precise compilation of the genealogy, as well as accurate ascertainment of medical information."

As he leaves the lecture hall, a gentleman approaches and introduces himself as Dr. Thomas Warthin, Aldred Warthin's son. The greying Veteran's Hospital physician says, "My father was extremely committed to Family G and was devoted to them to the end. I wish you the best of luck with your work."

Buoyed by this encounter, Lynch vows to continue his efforts. After being denied a grant from the National Institutes of Health,

America's leading government agency in biomedical research, Henry obtains funding from a host of private sources so he can outfit an RV with medical equipment and instruments for his next trip to Michigan. Driving from town to town, he and Krush administer questionnaires and take skin and blood samples from as many members of Family G as are willing.

"Cancer Family 'G' Revisited: 1895–1970" is published in the journal *Cancer* in June 1971.

Where Aldred Warthin had once written about "inferior stock," Lynch and Krush now present "a genetic reinvestigation" that squarely identifies the family as a clear representation of "cancer family syndrome." They also put forth the idea that there may be a distinct genotype for Family G, but add that, to date, "A dearth of identifying markers makes any attempt to predict incidence extremely difficult, since the diagnosis at this time must be based solely upon detailed family studies." As a gesture of thanks, Lynch and Krush send a family register to every participant in the study:

> We dedicate this "Family G" Register to all those wonderful family
> members who have so kindly assisted us by providing genealogical
> information and to all those who have offered to assist us in our
> research studies. Together we hope that all of your and our efforts will
> lead to a better understanding of hereditary factors in tumors.

When Sally's register arrives, she slowly thumbs through its pages until she finds her branch of the family tree. Her children are missing because she'd chosen not to give the researchers their names. *Maybe when they're older,* she thinks.

Her youngest daughter squeals through the house, chasing after one of her brothers. She has just turned three. Knowing the curly-headed imp's tendency for sticky fingers, Sally places the register in the bottom drawer of her dresser for safekeeping.

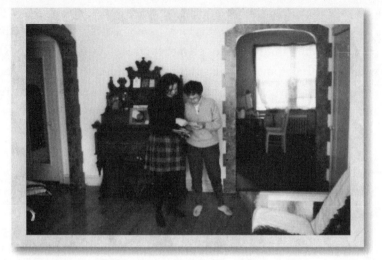

31.

A Heart Whose Love Is Innocent

Chicago, Illinois, 1995

It's after midnight and I'm sitting on the floor of a small, one-bedroom apartment, surrounded by crooked stacks of cardboard boxes. *Dishes. Books. Bedding. Books. Kitchen wares, CDs, bathroom stuff. Books.* I'd unpacked the Kid's things first, so he could fall asleep in his old bed in a new room in a city his mother doesn't really know. He's two years old.

What am I doing? I think, as I try to remember which box holds the hex keys I'll need to assemble the second-hand futon frame that's to serve as both our living-room couch and my bed.

The best I can.

I'd spent the past two years in flux, my heart pinballing between happiness and despair. I'd supported Brian when he'd needed me, stayed out of his way when he'd refused help. I'd bent over backwards to make sure that whatever time he spent with the Kid and me was relaxed, even fun. I'd never asked him to change a diaper, do the laundry or cook a meal. It'd been easier that way. Until it hadn't.

Not long after the baby's first birthday, I'd re-enrolled in school, hoping to finish my graduate degree. My former mentor had sent me an article with a note that'd simply read: "Thesis." It'd been the nudge I'd needed, academically and emotionally.

The article had featured a baritone named Will Parker, who'd been blackballed in the 1980s from the Metropolitan Opera because of his HIV-positive status. Unwilling to give up his life's work, Will had remade his career by becoming a musician-activist in the midst of the AIDS crisis.

After noticing that AIDS fundraisers within the music community largely featured classical music and little discussion about HIV or AIDS, he'd set out to change the culture by offering something different. Armed with poems written in response to the AIDS epidemic, he'd approached several composers and asked them to write art songs based on the texts. He'd called his project the AIDS Quilt Songbook, and made plans to perform it across the country, continually adding to it, song by song, musically mirroring the sewn panels that were constantly being added to the AIDS Quilt. Though Will died in spring 1993, months after the first concert, the project had lived on. My mentor had thought that I'd be the perfect person to document it.

As a first step, I'd sent questionnaires to the composers, poets and musicians involved in the project, hoping they'd be receptive to my plans for documenting the work. The Kid, of course, had come along for the ride. Seated in an aluminum-frame backpack meant for schlepping toddlers on long hikes, he'd babbled and played with my hair everywhere we went—library, concert hall, post office. In the evenings, he'd slept on an old sleeping bag on the floor next to my desk while I'd analyzed scores and typed page after page of notes. When I'd moved on to field research, he'd stayed with my parents, being spoiled by his "pa" and "lala" as I travelled from city to city in a beat-up VW van.

Everywhere I went (Minneapolis, Madison, Princeton, New York), I was greeted with open arms. Unified by Will's vision and love of life, the participants in the project had become a close-knit family, eager to share their experiences and their memories of Will. Several of the poets and composers were also HIV positive; I sometimes felt I was racing against time in seeking them out. With every interview and performance, I became more inspired, not just to chase after their stories, but to make sure I didn't waste a second of my life. One night, I was in the midst of a long, soul-searching conversation with Will's sister, Amy, when she'd mentioned that she needed to find a home for Will's dog, Nanook. I wound up volunteering to adopt the shepherd-husky mix. It felt like the "Will" thing to do.

Not long after I settled back home with Nanook and the Kid, Brian had gone off the deep end, again. He was moody, impatient and angry nearly all the time. I'd begged him to talk things through with a counsellor or a friend. My concern, as usual, had only served to make things worse.

"Just let me be fucked up!" he'd shouted. "I'm sick of this shit."

Me too, I'd thought, going silent. Our child was asleep in the next room. I didn't want him to hear us fight.

Nanook, who'd been trained to accompany Will through the streets of New York, put herself between me and Brian, barking at him.

"Fucking dog," he'd said, and kicked her hard in the ribs.

With a loud yelp, the frightened animal had scrambled to my side.

"You should go," I'd said, voice shaking. "Leave the house." I could hear the springs on our son's crib creak as he woke, and then his whimpering.

Brian had grabbed his keys and headed for the door, as Nanook, keeping a safe distance, trailed him, growling.

She didn't trust him anymore.

And neither did I.

I pick my way through the maze of boxes to look in on my son. He's sleeping peacefully, nestled in a twin bed that once belonged to my brother. Nanook is lying on a throw rug beside him, keeping guard. As the light from the hall spills into the room and across her face, her eyes shine.

"Good girl," I whisper, giving her a rub behind the ear.

It's taken us a while to get here, but we made it.

Chicago is a four-hour drive from where we used to live—if the traffic is good. Even though leaving had been the right choice, it has left a gaping hole in my heart. I'd accepted a temporary position at a small music college in the Windy City and Brian had taken a teaching gig back in Indiana just before I'd moved. At first, I'd thought that the time apart might do us good, but between our schedules and the distance between us, reconciling our differences now seemed unlikely.

Pulling my son's favourite blanket over his shoulders, I kiss the top of his head. I'd sewn the quilt for him when he was still in my womb, piecing it together from fabrics printed with constellations, old maps, jungle animals and a smiling yellow sun. It'd been my humble attempt to give him the world.

About a month after we moved, I drop the Kid and dog off at my parents, and drive to Toronto. There's a poet there connected to Will's songbook who I've been meaning to meet. Between single motherhood, a new job, and my washed-up marriage, completing my thesis has started to seem like a pipe dream. But giving up on it feels like giving up on myself, and I'm not willing to do that.

My first night in town, a friend invites me to come with him to a restaurant in Chinatown. "It's sort of a bon voyage for a guy who's heading off to school in Nova Scotia."

"I don't know," I say. "I wouldn't want to crash the party."

"It's just a bunch of guys eating short ribs and talking shit."

"Way to sell it."

"Please . . ."

"All right. But I can't stay long. I've got an early start tomorrow."

There are six of us altogether: me, my friend Earl, his brother Johnny, their friends Paul, Chachi and Ian (the one who's leaving for Nova Scotia in a week). We sit at a large round table in the back of a restaurant called Swatow, near a pair of swinging kitchen doors with rectangular portholes.

Johnny, who acts like an aspiring extra from a Tarantino film, orders a long list of items off the menu so we can eat family style. I half expect a bunch of mobsters to show up any minute to shake him down.

Hot and sour soup. Singapore vermicelli. Pork ribs with black bean sauce . . .

Once the food arrives, the guys take turns passing plates and razzing Ian about his decision to trade life in the Big Smoke for two years in a small university town. Between slurps of noodles, they exchange inside jokes and lines from old movies. Earl was right, it really is just five guys sucking on ribs and talking shit.

An hour in, I've had my fill. Putting my share of the bill on the table I turn to Earl and say, "I think I'm gonna call it a night."

"You can't go," he pleads. "All the plants are gonna die."

His friends crack up.

I don't.

"You get it, right?" he asks, thinking I've missed the joke. "It's Bill Murray, from *Stripes* . . ."

"Oh, I get it," I say. Without meaning to, he's cut too close to the bone. I can't help but think of Brian, and how he'd recently begged for another chance, insisting that he loved me, needed me, wanted me to stay. But he'd still refused to seek treatment. He'd said he was afraid they'd put him on some drug that would ruin his career as a musician. Grabbing my purse off the back of my chair, I say, "I really should go."

"If you stick around for a few more minutes," Earl says, "I'll give you a lift to your hotel."

Glancing at the door, I notice that a couple who's just entered the restaurant are dripping wet from a late summer downpour.

"Okay," I say, settling back in my chair. I'm not much for hailing cabs in the rain.

Sipping warm Coke through a straw stuck in the can, I watch the guys take turns giving Ian advice on how to score with women. He's being a really good sport.

"Honesty is the best way in," Johnny proclaims with cheesy swagger. "That, and a big schlong."

I sigh. I'm starting to regret not taking my chances with a cab.

"Dancing," Paul quickly offers, glancing my way. "If you're good together on the dance floor, then you'll be great together in bed."

Chachi, who's a swing dance instructor, wholeheartedly agrees.

"I rely on humour," Earl says, giving me a wink. "It's always worked for me."

"Has it?" I ask, and they laugh.

Ian finally speaks. "Poetry is the key."

"And a big schlong," Johnny teases.

Ignoring him, Ian goes on, "Language was invented for one reason, boys—to woo women." Eyes on me, he begins to recite: "She walks in beauty, like the night / Of cloudless climes and starry skies . . ."

I can't believe it. The adolescent prediction I'd scribbled on the back of a spiral notebook in 1983 is suddenly coming to life, and at the worst possible time.

Ian continues: "And all that's best of dark and bright / Meet in her aspect and her eyes—"

I raise my hand before he can finish the first stanza. "Please stop."

"Don't you like Byron?" Ian asks, looking a little hurt.

"I like him a lot," I say. "It's just . . ."

I push back from the table and stand up. "I have to go." Managing one shy glance at Ian, I add, "Best of luck."

Earl follows as I awkwardly skirt customers sliding out of booths and settling into chairs in the packed restaurant. Catching my arm as we reach the door, he asks, "What happened back there? Are you all right?"

The rain has stopped, so we head outside. "Just tired of all the guy talk." I move towards the crosswalk so I can hail a cab from the other side of the street. "You go back to the dinner. I'm fine."

We exchange hugs.

"For what it's worth," Earl says, squeezing my hand, "I think Ian likes you."

"That's ridiculous." *Impossible.* "He was just showing off."

Earl grins. "I think maybe *you* like him too."

Stepping off the curb, I wave the notion away. "That's the funniest thing you've said all night."

32.

Spit and Blood

Scots Bay, Nova Scotia, April 2018

Eldest Son has read through the instructions and filled out the necessary forms. Now all he needs to do is spit into a small plastic tube to seal the deal.

As saliva dribbles from his lips, we laugh at how ridiculous it is—this strange, awkward action he has to take in order to get an answer to one of the biggest questions of his life. For a moment, I'm five years old again, bursting into a fit of giggles as my brother Doug blows frothy spit bubbles. (This usually happened behind our mom's back while she was giving me a scolding.) Eldest Son is a lot like him—similar in looks and build, and with the same wicked sense of humour.

Securing the lid on the tube, he hands it to me. We'll need to pack it in its padded box, seal it in a large envelope and call the courier for pickup.

A string of odd thoughts pops into my head as I tuck the vial inside the foam casing that lines the box. People used to spit on their palms to make a pact; spit on their enemy's doorstep to cast a curse; spit on a freshly dug grave to show disrespect. Seamstresses, who'd accidentally pricked their fingers and left a tiny bloodstain, ran the thread they were using across their tongues and then poked the needle and thread through the red dot.

Sticking the box in the envelope, I ask, "How are you doing with all this?"

"Pretty good," he answers. "Considering."

"It's a bit of a roller-coaster ride, huh?"

"Yeah. But I'm pretty sure I'm positive."

"Oh, honey, no."

"It's okay, Mom. I really can't explain it. I just know I am."

I've been in his shoes. The closer you get to receiving *the* answer, the more your brain insists on doing strange math. Suddenly, every bond you share with those in your family who've had Lynch syndrome cancers becomes a flashing neon arrow pointed directly at your heart. Any closeness you have with them, in whatever form that might take, seems like evidence that you carry the same defective DNA.

Believing you're positive also serves as an act of self-preservation, because no matter the result, the fallout will be in your favour. If you're negative, your elation will be that much greater. If you're positive, you won't have so far to fall.

He'd learned to fly a plane before he could drive a car. He'd gone to university at seventeen, graduated at twenty-one. He'd spent a summer on the shores of the Aegean, and travelled near and far to gain a better understanding of the world and his art. The paintings and sculptures he creates are vibrant, joyous expressions of motion, colour and life. I can't bear the thought of anything ever standing in the way of his dreams.

Youngest Son joins us. He's a lot like his father—quiet, observant and always keen to find the best solution to any problem. His eyes go immediately to the medical pamphlets and letters from the lab that are strewn across the kitchen table.

"You can read all that stuff if you like," I tell him. "It's ours to keep."

I have filled him in on the basics of his brother's test, but as far as I know, he hasn't done a deep dive into figuring any of it out on his own. That's how he's always preferred to learn things—reading music, coding in several computer languages, knitting, speaking French. He's obsessively collected instruction manuals, pie charts and schematics since he was a toddler.

"Thanks," he says, thoughtfully considering a glossy trifold pamphlet titled: "Genetics and You." It weirdly complements his usual reading material: Isaac Asimov, Douglas Adams, Ray Bradbury, Terri Pratchett.

As Youngest Son reads, Eldest Son says, "The lab says they'll give a discount to any siblings or other relatives I refer to them for testing."

Youngest Son has just turned seventeen. He can be tested after his next birthday. "I'd like to do it as soon as possible," he says, placing the pamphlet back on the table. "I don't see any reason to wait."

"Okay," I say. "We'll get it done next year."

Eldest Son gives his brother a high five. "All right!"

God, I love my boys.

When I return to my research a few days later, I focus on the gap of time between Carl Weller's study at U of M in the 1930s and Henry Lynch's arrival in Ann Arbor in the mid-'60s.

It's during this time that family members become less traceable. In some branches they don't get married or have children; in other cases they simply drop out of sight. This family that was once so united by love and fate, is disappearing before my eyes. As I search through local newspaper articles, I note that family reunions come to an abrupt halt around this same time. The last mention of a reunion for Tillie's extended kin comes just before the group christening of her grandchildren in 1937.

I take comfort in the fact that her middle name, Anne, was given to four of her granddaughters, including my mother. To me it symbolizes hope as well as respect, like when a child is given the name of a saint in hopes that they'll be blessed with divine gifts. Tillie had lived through two cancers. To her kin she must've seemed like a walking miracle.

Revisiting Weller's report, I stare at the magnified images of my great-grandmother's two cancers. Phone in hand, I snap a few pictures of the grainy black-and-white slides, then try to sharpen their edges to bring them into focus. I've been following the University of Michigan's pathology department on social media, intrigued by the images they post for something they call #DailyDX, a pathologic guessing game, where people are invited to make observations about tissue samples from their labs. Wondering what they might make of my pics, I post them to my Twitter account and tag UMichPath.

Ami McKay @SideshowAmi
In April of 1936, pathologists Weller and Hauser from @
UMichPath presented a paper to the American Association for
Cancer Research regarding hereditary predisposition to cancer.
The report included this pair of "portraits" of my great-grand-
mother's cancers. She was the first member of her family to
undergo surgery and survive to live a long life.
#LynchSyndrome #memoir #DNA #FamilyG #pathology
#HistMed #genetics #genealogy

Staring at the screen, I wonder if anyone who currently works there has any idea of the role the institution played in my relatives' lives? (For better or for worse?)

I'd recently read that the Board of Regents had voted to remove the name of former president C.C. Little from a science building on Central Campus. The committee report clearly states that it was due in large part to Little's promotion of eugenics, a stance that led to serious negative consequences in the lives of many people.

A few minutes after posting Tillie's slides, I get a response from @UMichPath.

Michigan Pathology @UMichPath
This is an amazing piece of history! We're so proud of Drs
Hauser and Weller. Thank you for sharing!

Ami McKay @SideshowAmi
Who should I contact to discuss the history of the pathology
department at U of M?

I've no idea if they have anything left relating to Family G, but I figure it can't hurt to ask.

A direct message from their social media account leads to an email contact, which in turn leads to the anatomic pathology office manager, Nancy Fritzemeier.

NF:

I am happy to help, but it will be tricky since the record keeping is pretty sketchy. I am sure folks didn't comprehend the volumes of testing that would be possible 90 years later!

I have pathology reports that go back to 1925; the records are kept on a CD with no relatable naming convention, so we have to open each PDF to see if it matches your relatives. Can you provide dates of birth?

And so begins a flurry of messages between Nova Scotia and Ann Arbor on a sunny spring afternoon.

I send Nancy dates for Pauline and Tillie, as well as all the information I've got on the slides that appear in Weller's report: 3526-W, 1-X, 4987-AI, 5078-AI, 371-AI. The strings of numbers and letters don't make much sense to me, but I'm hoping that they'll mean something to her.

NF:

I have the path reports for your great grandmother's cases and we are working on retrieving the tissue blocks from our offsite storage. It's been extremely helpful to have the reference numbers.

The thought that Pauline's and Tillie's tissue still exists in some storage facility in Michigan makes me weepy. The two sisters, or at least small parts of them, may soon meet again. And I may be able to see both of them for the first time in colour.

As I wrap up my work for the day, Eldest Son calls to say that his sample has arrived at the lab and that he should get his results on May 14.

After we hang up, I mark it on the calendar. May 14 is the day after Mother's Day. *Positive or negative, which will he be?* Either way, he is, I am, we are, the sum of many things.

I've been thinking a lot about his "knowing" that he's positive, and wondering about the nature of memory across generations. I've been an aspiring genealogist since my childhood, chasing Family G's history for as long as I can remember. Pauline and Tillie now feel more real to me than some people I've known my entire life. I suppose that's why it puzzles me that some members of my family are completely unaware of this part of our collective past. Knowing the very real consequences of ignoring our lineage of disease, I find it even more baffling to discover that some relatives actively choose to dismiss it. Is it easier to live an unexamined life? I wouldn't know.

When I was young, my older sister, Lori, was terrified of the dark. She kept a lamp on in the room we shared, all night, every night, until she got married and moved away at eighteen. The base of the lamp was a porcelain carousel horse with a striped pole coming out its back that held the fixture for the bulb and the shade. Staring at the yellowing shade long past my bedtime, I'd imagine what it might feel like to die.

My brother Doug says he can't imagine things when he closes his eyes. I tell him I see too much when I do.

Maybe my son does know.

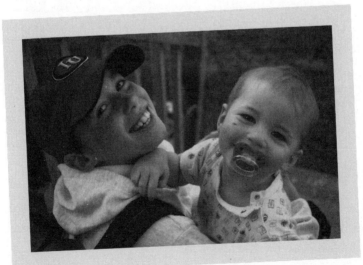

Eldest Son and Youngest Son

33

Garden of Dreams

Scots Bay, Nova Scotia, February 2000

As I stand in the kitchen of an old farmhouse on the Bay of Fundy, I can barely see the floor for all the half-empty boxes scattered around the room. *Books. Dishes. Pots and pans. Books. Bathroom stuff, Glassware. Cleaning supplies. Books.*

The Kid skirts past me, cutting through the cardboard maze with a gawky puppy nipping at his heels. They skitter down the hallway and run upstairs—all sneakers, paws and tail wagging. The Kid is now six years old; Sophie, the pup, is nine months. The house has stood for well over a century, a bit worse for wear, but stubborn in her bones.

The mud-room door swings open as Ian delivers another box to my arms. "For you, Mrs. McKay."

"Thank you, Mr. McKay."

I add it to the rest. *More books.*

It's taken us five years to get here, but we're home.

After that rainy night in Toronto when I'd run out the doors of Swatow trying to escape fate, I'd returned to Chicago and focused all my attention on the Kid and work.

Trading in my temporary job at the music college for a permanent teaching position, I spend the next four years as a music instructor at a private school for the arts. When the Kid graduates from preschool, he attends kindergarten in a room downstairs from my office.

Our neighbourhood is a sketchy mix of crack dealers, gang-bangers, college students and artists, but our apartment is close to the El Train. The Kid and I ride the train to school most days, crooning along with the singing conductor as he'd belts out each stop. "This is Loyola. Loy-ohhhhhhhh-laaaaah!" is his morning refrain. "Sher-i-dan. Your next stop is Sher-ihhhhh-daaaan," is our welcome home.

On warm summer nights we throw the windows open to catch a breeze off the lake and the sound of Harry Caray leading the crowd at Wrigley Field during the seventh inning stretch. "For it's one, two, three strikes you're out, at the old ball game!" The Kid falls asleep with the Goodyear blimp circling overhead like an enormous mechanical firefly blinking, G-O C-U-B-B-I-E-S !

Life is as good as I can make it, but it's also exhausting. In addition to money always being tight, there's the emotional and physical toll of doing everything alone. My only nearby friend is my old university roommate, Dawn, who lives an hour's drive away. We visit each other whenever we can, but I spend most of my evenings and weekends lonely for adult conversation.

The summer I turn thirty, I plant a tiny garden in my North Side neighbourhood, hoping to make one small corner of the city a little brighter. Without asking anyone's permission, I adopt a five-by-five tree square that sits along the sidewalk across the street from my apartment. Devoting an entire weekend and a coffee can of spare change to the project, the Kid and I collect all the trash from the square; edge the tiny plot with old bricks we find in the alley behind our building; plant mums, impatiens and ageratums around the tree; carry plastic milk jugs full of water down the three flights of stairs from our apartment; and mulch the whole thing with a layer of cedar chips. For a finishing touch, we tie a ribbon with a note around the tree's trunk featuring the Kid's original art. Sunday evening we stand at the windows of our apartment, watching sparrows hop around the base of the tree pecking for bugs. For a moment, I even dare to daydream aloud, "maybe we'll plant tulip bulbs in the fall and hang a small bird feeder in the tree's branches during the winter."

The following morning I come downstairs to discover a man standing in the little garden, urinating against the tree, my tree. Once he finishes relieving himself and stumbles away, I cross the street to inspect for damage. Two of the four mums we'd planted are missing, and one of the bricks from the border is also gone. The passenger window of a car parked next to the tree is smashed, and the car's stereo, stolen. All that's left is a gaping hole with a few stray electrical wires. A brick, my brick, is lying on the passenger seat in a pile of broken glass.

At first, I blame these unfortunate events on urban life, believing that Chicago is just a mean, heartless place where much worse things happen every day. But in time, I realize that it isn't the city's fault, but mine. I keep making the mistake of planting my dreams in the wrong place.

Brian fares much better at moving on. He meets a lovely woman, joins the army and moves to South Carolina. I send him off with good wishes, hoping he's finally found a way of moving through the world that will make him happy. His interactions with the Kid are few and far between, but it seems to be a speed that he can handle.

Maybe, I think, *love just isn't in the cards for me.*

Evenings after the Kid goes to bed, I escape into an online chat room set up by my friend Earl in Toronto. He and his brother Johnny had started a small internet service provider, and they'd opened the chat room as a way for the ISP's users to meet. Giving myself a new name, I enjoy the freedom of conversing with people from around the world in complete anonymity. It's a convenient escape from the slog of daily life.

It's also how I cross paths again with Ian, only this time I don't run away. He's also chosen to use an alias, but it doesn't take long for me to figure out who he is. How many poetry-loving-education-students-from-Toronto-now-living-in-Nova Scotia could there be? Once I reveal my identity to him (and apologize for bolting from the restaurant) we quickly fall into a friendship that blossoms both in and out of the chat room.

We're soon acting like a pair of kids swapping notes in the back of class, only our exchanges are largely devoted to favourite authors, poets and philosophers. Occasionally we take stabs at giving each other relationship advice.

> She's never going to be what you need. You can't *fix* someone who doesn't want to change.

> You know he was no good for you, right? I say you're better off without him.

We look at the world in a similar way. We want the same things in life—home, family, honesty, true love—but neither of us possesses the courage to admit that we might be the other's ideal mate. The distance is too great, too difficult to overcome. I'm the girl no one wants for keeps.

On a frosty morning mid-October 1998, I decide to drive my car to school rather than take the train. I'm running late, so I quickly settle the Kid in the front passenger seat and snap his seat belt into place. My seat belt refuses to retract securely across my chest, and I don't have time to fix it. Sliding the belt's clip into the buckle, I let the belt flop off my shoulder and set off.

Two blocks later, a car comes barrelling down a side street, screams through a stop sign and smashes into the front of my vehicle. With crumpling metal and shattering glass, the windshield gives way and the rear-view mirror collides with my face. As my eyes swell shut, I reach out to my son. "Are you okay?" I ask, fearing the worst.

"I'm fine, Mommy," he answers, but I can hear panic in his voice.

"What's wrong?" I ask. "Are you hurt?"

"There's blood, Mommy," he sobs. "All over you."

Struggling to stay conscious, I hear someone opening the door on my side of the car. A woman with a calm, steady voice says, "There's an ambulance coming. You're going to be okay."

Sirens wail in the distance.

"What about my son?" I ask. "I can't see anything. Is he all right?"

"There's not a scratch on him. He's fine."

It's the last thing I hear.

Two weeks later, after I've been released from hospital, my phone rings late at night.

Fumbling for the receiver I answer with a groggy, "Hello?"

"Ami?" a man's voice asks.

I can't place it.

"It's me, Ian."

"Oh, gosh, hi," I say in complete surprise. Neither of us ever has enough money for long distance calls. It's been ages since I've heard his voice.

"Is it too late to talk?"

My face has started to heal, but my brain has suffered a terrible knocking. I'm still having trouble focusing on things, like music scores, computer screens and conversations. I haven't been online since the accident, which means I haven't been in touch with Ian, either. "No, it's fine," I say. "It's really good to hear from you."

"Earl told me about your accident. How are you doing?"

"It's slow going, but I'll be all right. I just have to take it easy. The doctor ordered me off work for a month, so I'm pretending it's a paid vacation."

He says, "If you ever need a place to get away, you're welcome to come visit me. No strings attached."

"Thanks," I say, a little shocked by his offer. "I'll keep that in mind."

One month later, with the Kid on a trip with his paternal grandfather to see Brian, I get on a plane to Halifax. It seems like the perfect time to visit a kind-hearted friend in a place I've never been.

And it is. Within minutes of my arrival, I find I've never felt so at ease, at home or in love in my entire life. And, to my astonishment, Ian feels the same way. What once seemed impossible is suddenly meant-to-be. By the end of the first night, Ian has recited the Byron poem in full, and my faith in magic has been restored. Between the tides and starry skies, we make plans to start a life together.

Not long after my trip to Nova Scotia, Ian comes to stay with me and the Kid in Chicago. It's clear from the start that they're meant to be father and son.

Gaining my mother's approval is harder. When she finally meets Ian, she gives him the third degree, peppering him with warnings like "You understand this is a package deal" and "You know that kid and his mom are precious cargo." Pointing her finger at him, she asks, "This is forever, right?"

Dad and I stand in the kitchen, listening. "Poor fella," he whispers. "But I'm rooting for him."

"Me too," I whisper back.

Ian gives Mom an honest, forthright response. "I can't control the future, but if I have any say in the matter, then, yes, it's forever."

"Good," Mom says with a wink. "You got the answer right."

With my parents' blessing, we are married in a courthouse in Kings County, Nova Scotia, by a judge, who for unknown reasons has a black eye. After saying our legal "I dos" in front of him, we exchange our own vows on a cliff overlooking the sea, with a pasture full of cows behind us, bells jangling around their necks as they graze. It's all the fanfare we need.

The house we're now settling into isn't far from that spot. It, too, looks over the sea. We've got big hopes for this place and for what lies ahead, and although it's the dead of winter, I've already chosen a spot to plant a garden. Maybe the key to everything—love, happiness, dreams, magic—is giving it room to grow.

Tonight my son will fall asleep in a new country; in a place unlike anywhere else he's ever lived. Rather than hearing a lullaby of sirens, car horns and the rattle of the El, he'll drift off to the rhythmic pulse of the tide churning stones on the beach—the voice of the moon.

What will he dream of?

Who will he become?

No matter what the future holds, *this* is home.

34.

The Problem with Humans

Johns Hopkins University, Baltimore, Maryland, February 2000
An article in the February 17 edition of *Nature* states:

> The problem with humans, at least from the perspective of genetic
> diagnostics, is that they have two copies of each of their chromo-
> somes (diploidy). Mutations in one copy of a chromosome pair can
> therefore be obscured by the normal sequence present on the other
> copy of the chromosome. Here we describe a way to overcome this
> problem and expose the masked mutation by converting the human
> chromosome complement to a haploid state through fusion to a
> novel recipient cell line. This approach can significantly increase the
> sensitivity of genetic tests.

In other words, the team of genetic researchers that Henry Lynch
had so enthusiastically spoken of to my mother in the early 1990s has
finally developed a way to tease out the defect in her DNA that leads
to cancer. It's taken seven years of exhaustive work, much of it done in
a laboratory housed in a former strip-mall supermarket, but the causal
mutation for Family G has been found.

Run by co-principal investigators Dr. Bert Vogelstein and Dr. Ken
Kinzler, the lab has eighteen post-doctoral and five pre-doctoral students on its staff, many of whom refer to Vogelstein as "the Jedi Master."
It's his relaxed manner and straightforward philosophy that sets the
tone for their work. He never pits students against one another to

solve the same problem, but encourages an atmosphere of collaboration where everyone plays a part. This is why it's fast becoming one of the most important oncology labs in the world.

Twice a week, they all eat lunch together in a large conference room and discuss their respective projects. On Tuesdays, the same room is converted into a practice space for the lab's in-house rock band, Wild Type. Vogelstein plays keyboards, Kinzler plays drums, and other members of the research team fill out the ensemble at various times.

Vogelstein appreciates his students as much as they revere him. They remind him of the importance of refusing to believe something can't be done.

Shortly after Vogelstein and others had discovered the linkage between mutations in the MSH2 gene and colorectal cancer in the early '90s, Vogelstein reached out to Lynch to say he'd like to "see if this gene, or related genes are the culprits in the families you've been painstakingly collecting." Aware that Lynch's data on Family G spanned a century, he was convinced that his team and Lynch's research would make a perfect match.

Lynch had a freezer full of DNA from the families he'd been studying, many members with what he was now calling hereditary nonpolyposis colorectal cancer, or HNPCC, because of the disease's tendency to present in the form of a large tumour in the colon rather than a proliferation of polyps. (The name would soon be changed to "Lynch syndrome" by Lynch's colleague C. Richard Boland, in an effort to honour Henry's efforts and accommodate the myriad of cancers associated with the syndrome.)

Lynch was overjoyed by the prospect of collaborating with Vogelstein's team at Johns Hopkins. If Vogelstein could identify the exact problem with Family G's DNA, he'd finally have the genetic needle-in-a-haystack he'd been hoping for all these years. It would prove once and for all that cancer can in fact be caused by inherited genetic factors; that knowledge, in turn, would save lives.

So began the hunt.

❧

Initially, several of the non–Family G samples Lynch sent readily present with visible mutations after Vogelstein's team puts them through analysis. Others didn't—most notably the sample from Family G, my mother's.

Month after month, year after year, the mutation responsible for the family's cancers eluded the team's intensive efforts to identify it. Even after putting the Family G sample through every conventional testing technique available to them, they still had no answers. This frustrated Vogelstein to no end. Of all the DNA they had, why wouldn't this one reveal its secret? He knew something must be present given the sample was, in his words, "from the family that started everything."

Rather than give up, he and his team decided to approach the problem a different way.

First, they recommitted to the idea that a mutation must be present.

Second, they decided that if it can't be seen by conventional analysis, they simply needed to invent another, more robust technique for detecting it.

In the end, they settled on playing a high-stakes game of genetic hide-and-seek. And that changed everything.

Assuming the mutation is there but not identifiable by available means, they need to invent a better way to "seek."

Every person has two copies of each gene—one from the mother and one from the father. In order to discuss differences or variations in a gene's pairing, biologists refer to the individual copies as "alleles." In traditional DNA sequencing, a researcher sees both alleles for each gene they're examining simultaneously. If, say, a deletion has removed the entire allele that came from the mother, the researcher will still see the unaffected allele from the father and think everything looks normal. Long story short, a normal allele can mask a deletion, hiding the mutation.

So the researchers asked: *What if we could separate a pair of alleles so we could look at them individually?*

The idea was deceptively simple yet technologically vexing. It had never been done.

For the next three years, a post-doc from Beijing named Hai Yan devoted himself to solving the problem. Working day and night, Yan made many attempts at perfecting a process he called "conversion"—a technique whereby a gene's diploid state can be changed to haploid in order to reveal a deleterious mutation. His girlfriend worried about his taxing schedule and his constant frustration over not making progress in the lab. Yan worried that her parents wouldn't think him successful enough to be a suitable match for their daughter.

In 1999, he made yet another attempt to get it right, this time through the use of a special strain of mouse cells meant to stabilize the transferred human chromosomes. On a sunny summer day, after a paintball game with other research fellows, Yan came back to the lab to check on his work. Paint still on his face, he stared at a funny band in the sequencing gel. Vogelstein, who was at his side, gave him a high five. The veil had been lifted. A hundred-year puzzle, solved.

Yan immediately called his girlfriend to tell her that they'd just made an important discovery in human health history. He then asked her permission to meet with her family. "Yes," she said, "but don't brag about your work, they already know you're a good man. This only proves you can do something important." They were married within a year.

Vogelstein's first call was to Henry Lynch to give him the good news. The lab's innovation not only provided Family G with the answer they'd been waiting for, it would also end up doing the same for many other families whose genetic cancer mutations had been hidden from view. The technique was solid and improved the sensitivity of the test from between 70 and 80 percent to close to 100 percent. The notion that cancer had no genetic link could now be put to rest. Lynch's work had been validated beyond a shadow of a doubt.

Pauline Gross's wishes had finally come true. Never again would a member of her family have to guess at their fate. By the prick of a needle or a spot of spit, they'll know for sure.

Stories hold
our cure.

—Hannah Gadsby

Hope. Trust. Dream.

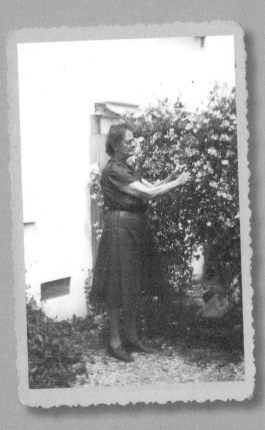

Previous page: Tillie picking sweet peas

35·

Family Reunion

University of Michigan, Ann Arbor, March 2000
My mother enters a large conference room in the university's Comprehensive Cancer Center. The building is situated on a road that eases along a verdant bend in the Huron River, just a ten-minute walk from her great-aunt Pauline's final resting place in Forest Hill. Once she's inside the door, she's greeted by a pair of members from the research team who are hosting today's event. The lab-coat-wearing duo check her name off a list, give her an envelope filled with documents and hand her a name tag.

HELLO

MY NAME IS

SALLY

She sticks the tag to her sweater, over her heart—marking the spot where she'd often placed her hand to show allegiance, respect, empathy, gratitude, sorrow. Scanning the room she looks for familiar faces. Aside from the dozen or so medical personnel in attendance, everyone else is kin. This isn't just a medical conference, it's a family reunion.

"Mom." Her eldest daughter, Lori, catches up to her. "They've got bagels and pastries and coffee. You want anything?"

Sally glances at the spread on the other side of the room. It looks enticing enough, surprisingly so, which causes her to feel strangely empty-handed—she has no sugar cream pie or potato salad or foil-wrapped casserole to add to the feast. "Just coffee for me," she answers. "Black." Her voice creaks from nervous cigarette consumption and lack of sleep. She knows she should quit smoking, and God knows she's tried, but on the way here with Lori and Lori's daughter, Anna, one cigarette had turned into half a pack, and then she'd taken a wrong turn. When she'd stopped to ask a security guard for directions to the cancer centre, smoke had billowed out the car window in his face.

Her granddaughter had tried and failed to stifle her laughter from the back seat. *Anna's such a good sport*, Sally thinks. At nineteen, the affable young woman is her eldest grandchild, and the only one old enough to come to the conference.

Settling into a front row seat, Sally scans the people lingering around the food table. Their faces are older, leaner, bearing the toll of time and cancer, but flashes of familiarity remain from encountering them at long-ago funerals, weddings, family picnics, and photographs stuck inside Christmas cards. *Could that woman be Kit's daughter? How old would she be now? Thirty-five? Forty? How long has it been since I've seen her? Fifteen, twenty years? I should've been better about keeping in touch. I should've called more often, tried harder.*

Suzanne, the cousin she'd been closest to, had died seven years earlier of heart failure at sixty-two. Sally is now sixty-six, and edging up on her ninth year post-cancer. She'd like to think that she's seen the last of it, but she knows that's not how this works. *Not when it comes to cancer. Not for us.*

Catching the attention of a doctor who's walking past, she asks, "How many family members are you expecting here today?"

"Around thirty," the ginger-haired man answers. He's got a freckled forehead and a kind smile. "Give or take."

"Thanks," Sally says, wishing all of her kids had agreed to come.

"Thank *you* for being here," he says.

The meeting had been arranged by Dr. Lynch's lab at Creighton University in conjunction with a research team from the University of Michigan. Since more family members still live in Michigan than anywhere else, they'd chosen to hold the event in Ann Arbor. Invitations for the "Family Information Session" had been sent out months in advance along with the offer that for the first time, genetic testing would be available. On the RSVP card, people were to check one:

❏ YES, I PLAN ON DONATING A BLOOD SAMPLE FOR GENETIC TESTING.
❏ NO, I DO NOT PLAN ON DONATING A BLOOD SAMPLE FOR GENETIC TESTING.

A far cry from choosing "Chicken" or "Vegetarian."
There hadn't been any option that'd applied to Sally's particular situation, so she'd checked yes and then written in the margin, "I've already donated blood and tissue samples, but I'm happy to give more if you need it."

She watches as the doctor she'd spoken to earlier walks to the front of the room to make an announcement. "I'm afraid Dr. Lynch is stuck in traffic, but he should be here soon. Thank you for your patience."

Sally's niece Holly, her brother's second oldest daughter, comes up to her to say hello with her older sister, Heather, and younger brother, Ashley, in tow. It's clear Ashley would rather be someplace else.

He looks more like my uncle Bud every year.
"Hey, schnicklefritz," Sally says, giving Holly a warm hug.
"Hey, Aunt Saucie," Holly replies, kissing Sally's cheek.
After exchanging affectionate greetings with the siblings, Sally asks, "Where's the rest of your clan?"

"It's just us for today," Holly says. "I tried my best, but I couldn't get any more takers." Her niece had been hoping to get all five of her siblings to attend and had been calling them repeatedly for weeks.

"Well, they're missing out," Sally says. "If the people in our family had had this test before, think of all the suffering and lives it could have saved. By being here, you're honouring your ancestors."

Sally doesn't admit the heaviness she feels in her own heart over the absence of three of her four children. Larry had told her not to worry about it. "Give them time. They're smart, responsible adults. They'll come around." But this isn't like waiting for your kid to come to their senses over wasting their allowance or hanging out with the wrong crowd. This is life or death.

Her two eldest, Skip and Doug, are now forty-five and forty-four. They have solid careers, families and mortgages. Skip says he needs more information and time before he can decide. Doug worries that his test results might get into the wrong hands, causing him to be dismissed from his job or to lose his health insurance.

"They've told me it's all confidential," Sally had stressed.

"But how can you know that for sure?"

"I trust the process. I trust Dr. Lynch."

Sally's youngest daughter has just moved to Canada, so flying home for the meeting hadn't made sense. At least she'd shown some interest in learning more about the test. "Have them send me the forms and I'll look into what needs to be done on my end."

"Will do."

Sally isn't convinced that she will follow through, though.

They'd all seen what she'd gone through with her cancer. Why wasn't that enough? She feels as if she's walking a tightrope, barely able to find her balance between her love for her children and her trust in their judgment.

Last week she'd called Henry's assistant, Ali, in a panic. "If my children don't come to the session, can they still get the test?"

"Yes, of course," the young woman had promised. "We're more than happy to arrange it."

At least there's that.

When Dr. Lynch finally arrives, his hair is a bit dishevelled and his clothes are wrinkled, but his voice is steady and clear. "I'd like to begin by thanking you for your willingness to help me and my team. With your participation we'll be able to help not only your family, but countless others around the world." He never wastes any time in getting down to business. Sally has always appreciated that about him.

The doctor clicks his controller and an image of the family tree pops up on a large screen. It dates back to Pauline and Tillie's grandfather, who died in 1856 from stomach cancer. "Today, there are nine hundred and twenty-nine descendants from the progenitor first mentioned in Warthin's 1913 study," Lynch says and explains that occurrences of cancer are indicated by blackened circles and squares. The chart looks as if it's been used for target practice at a shooting range.

Even with her knowledge of the family's history of cancer, Sally finds it sobering to see it all laid out before her, especially as Henry rattles off a grim list of statistics.

The number of cancers.

The various types.

The ages of those affected.

The lives lost.

He doesn't assign any names to the dozens of dark marks that dot the chart, but Sally knows who they are.

"Thirty-five percent of all cancers in Family G come from Branch I, even though this particular branch is only 12 percent of the total family. Kindred from Branch I also tend to present with cancer at an earlier age." Sally can draw a direct line through Branch I—*from Kathrina, to Tillie, to Alice, to me.*

As she lets the numbers sink in, Dr. Lynch speaks of progress and the future. He tells them that in the past three decades, he's been fairly successful in educating others about familial cancer syndromes. A growing number of medical professionals are now familiar with his research—gastroenterologists, endoscopists, pathologists, genetic counsellors, laboratory investigators, general practitioners. Because of this, protocols have been developed to support increased surveillance for Family G and other families with similar syndromes. For Sally's family, more colonoscopies, endoscopies and endometrial biopsies have meant earlier detection and fewer deaths from cancer. Several laboratories have added to the growing body of research by establishing tumour registries around the world.

"And now," Henry says, "genetic testing will, at long last, make clinical diagnosis possible for Family G."

As she listens to him outline the discovery that'd been made in Bert Vogelstein's laboratory with a single sample from a member of Family G, Sally swears he's looking straight at her.

She feels gratitude in this moment, and hope too, though both feel bittersweet. While she'd gladly given permission for her tissues to be used for research, and she'd considered it her duty to help others, the realization of what it means to carry "the gene" is starting to sink in. If the confirmed sample from Family G was hers, then there's a fifty-fifty chance she's passed the mutation on to her children, and they in turn, on to theirs.

Once Dr. Lynch has finished his presentation, the team invites individual family members into separate rooms for private consultations.

Sally sits with Anna while Lori takes her turn.

"Are you nervous?" she asks the girl as she squeezes her hand.

"Yes."

"Just try to relax, sweetheart. Be honest, tell the truth. Don't forget they're there to help you."

Lori looks shaken when she returns.

"Are you all right?" Sally asks.

Sitting on the other side of her, Lori whispers. "I thought they were just going to collect some blood and discuss the study, but it turned out to be more intense."

Sally doesn't believe in pretending something doesn't exist. "How so?" she asks, refusing to whisper back.

"For starters, they asked some pretty personal questions. They wanted to know if I'd consider having a hysterectomy if I test positive for the gene. Even though I'm perfectly healthy."

A nurse calls Anna's name.

Lori catches her daughter's arm as the girl moves past. "Are you sure you still want to do this? I'll understand if you've changed your mind."

"I'll be fine, Mom," Anna says. "Don't worry."

Lori bites her thumbnail as she watches her daughter walk away.

"She's a smart girl," Sally says. "They'll put the information in front of her and she'll take it in as best she can. We'll see her through the rest."

A few minutes later, Sally's name is called.

"Sarah Bartz . . ." Sarah Anne, Sally, Sal. Granddaughter, daughter, sister, wife, mother of four, grandmother of six, cancer survivor, medical subject.

She walks into the room and sits across from a genetic counsellor at a table.

"Am I the one?" she asks.

"Pardon?" the nurse replies.

"The member of Family G whose gene showed up on the test."

The nurse stares at the paperwork in front of her on the table. "If you take part in today's study, you'll have your results in a couple of months."

Sally points at the papers. "I'm sure you can see that I've already had cancer. And you probably also know that my tissue samples were sent to Baltimore. If you already have the answer, then I'd like to know today. It's my right."

"There are emotional repercussions, Mrs. Bartz, that I'd like you to consider."

"I'm more than happy to hear you out, but I'm not leaving until I get an answer."

By the time she walks out of the building, she'll have it. *Yes.*

She doesn't think about herself. Doesn't wallow in self-pity or guilt. What's most important to her now is finding the best way to help her children cope with whatever lies ahead. She can't fix their DNA, but she can do everything in her power to get all four of them to take the test. She's already thinking of what she'll say to them, already forming an argument in her head. *Knowledge is power.*

36.

Signs

Scots Bay, Nova Scotia, April 2018

I'm fourth in line at the local pharmacy, waiting for a morning blood draw. Today's needle stick is in service of my annual blood work-up for Lynch syndrome. Early detection is key. It reminds me of something my dad used to say: "You can save yourself a lot of grief just by checking the oil in your car."

My GP is still chasing after the cause of my heart murmur. The results from my twenty-four-hour blood pressure test had turned out fine, but she'd decided to send me in for an echocardiogram.

Yesterday morning, I'd lain on my back in a hospital bed while a tech had held an ultrasound sensor to various spots on my chest. The test had been painless and brief, but I'd been shocked to hear the sound of my heart glugging away over a speaker in the darkened room. I've no idea what a heart is supposed to sound like in that setting, but mine had sounded more like the *boom-chick-a-boom* of a burlesque drummer than the steady *lub-dub* I'd heard through the stethoscope Mom kept in the back of a bathroom cabinet in my childhood home. I used to pull it out from behind a tangle of hairdryer and curling iron cords, and listen to my own heart while waiting for the bathtub to fill. I'd loved the isolation it'd provided, the sensation of perfect loneliness.

At least with yesterday's echocardiogram, no doctor had come rushing into the room from some distant corner of the hospital. The tech hadn't once gasped in horror. Because of this, I've decided to assume everything is fine, until I hear different.

The visiting nurse at the pharmacy calls the next person in line. I'm now number three. It seems as if some part of me is always under the scrutiny of a medical expert.

The lab in charge of testing Eldest Son's DNA had recently contacted him with a request for additional information about my specific mutation. I'd sent them copies of every report, chart and file I'd had on hand. I'm once again worried about whether their testing process is rigorous enough. I'd grilled the lab tech pretty hard when I'd spoken with her over the phone, but the more I learn about the stealthy nature of my particular mutation, the more I wonder if I've sent my son in the wrong direction. Is it possible they'll get a wrong result? A false positive or a false negative: which is worse?

Sometimes I wonder if my own test results could be wrong, though the rest of the time I'm wondering when cancer's going to rear its ugly head. Occasionally Ian reminds me that it's statistically possible to have the gene and never get cancer, but that proposition feels far-fetched to me. It's actually easier for me to imagine that I've unwittingly been pulled into a terrible social experiment where the "results" of my genetic test were faked so "researchers" can monitor the long-term effects of my believing I have a defective gene.

I can't recall my mother ever letting her imagination run wild like this. We talked at length on several occasions about her attitude and feelings about cancer and Lynch syndrome. She'd always seemed focused and determined, and doggedly set on all of her children getting tested, especially after Lori's results had come back negative. The relief she'd felt about Lori, and therefore all three of Lori's children also being mutation-free (Lynch syndrome doesn't skip generations), had given her the energy and resolve she'd needed to push harder on the rest of us. Although I'd been the next to submit to the test, I regret every minute she'd had to wait while I'd made up my mind. The regret is doubly keen now that I'm in her shoes.

The nurse calls the next person in line, and a woman who appears to be in her mid-seventies steps forward. There's no door between the waiting area and the nurse's station, so I can hear the woman and the nurse making small talk as I wait.

"Nice weather today," the nurse says. "And it's about time too, don't you think?"

"Yes," the woman agrees with a sharp uptake of breath. The Nova Scotia inhaled affirmative. A linguistic beauty mark that distinguishes her from "come from aways" like me. I've lived here for eighteen years, I'm now a Canadian citizen, and I'm still trying to get it right.

"Is it still sunny out there?" the nurse asks. The space she's using is a windowless room in the back of the drugstore.

"It was when I come in," the woman answers. "And warm enough this morning to sit and watch the birds from my back porch."

I hear the snap of an elastic band as the nurse says, "I like to watch the birds too. Lately there's been a cardinal that shows up around suppertime every evening, out my back window."

"Oh, that's really special!" the woman says.

"Make a fist," the nurse instructs. "This'll just be a little pinch."

The woman keeps talking through the prick of the needle. "Seeing a cardinal means someone you've lost is coming for a visit to say hello."

"That's such a lovely thought," the nurse says. "I've never heard of it before."

"Oh, yes," the woman says. "It's old wisdom. It's been around a long time. My grandmother taught it to me when I was a child."

"Isn't that something?"

"And now you know it too, so when you see that bird again, you can make the connection. Maybe to someone who's been on your mind."

As the nurse finishes the woman's blood draw, it's all I can do not to cry. My mother had told me the same thing when we'd spotted a cardinal in her aunt Doris's garden after she'd died. Mom believed in magic—in keeping the heart and mind and senses open to gifts left in your path. A feather on the sidewalk or a special song played on the radio, could easily be a message from a higher power—call it God, or the Universe, or Spirit, or Serendipity. The "thing" that got sent was never the point. It was the connection formed between it and you. As Mom used to say, "The story your heart makes in that moment is the magic."

Yesterday I was missing her so desperately that I was talking to her out loud as I drove home from the hospital. I suspect she heard me.

Before I can talk myself out of the notion, the nurse comes into the waiting room and says, "Next."

Sometimes, for a moment, everything is just as you need it to be. The memories of such moments live in the heart, waiting for the time you need to think of them, if only to remind yourself that for a short while, everything had been fine, and might be so again.

—Ami McKay, *The Virgin Cure*

37.

The Birth House

Scots Bay, Nova Scotia, July 2000

Two boxes sit next to each other on my kitchen table—one metal, one cardboard. Both are about the size of a loaf of bread, each labelled with a sticky note that says: "For Ami." My parents have just driven the 2,400 kilometres from Indiana in a gas-guzzling SUV pulling an RV travel trailer they call "the Ritz." They'd purchased the RV a few years back so they could celebrate Dad's retirement with an epic road trip to Alaska.

Dad says that driving to Nova Scotia was a breeze.

"Except for Montreal," Mom teases.

"Even Montrealers don't like driving there," I say.

Mom nods. "We'll be taking a different route home."

Within an hour they've both fallen into full-on parental mode—Dad tromping through the backyard with Ian and the Kid to make measurements for a new jungle gym they're going to build together; Mom snooping through my fridge and kitchen cupboards so we can plan our meals for the next three weeks.

After taking an inventory of the empty canning jars I've got in the pantry, she decides we need to make jam. "If the weather's good tomorrow, we'll go strawberry picking."

"Sure," I say, "that sounds fun." I don't mean it.

I'd been hoping she and Dad might take a day or two to relax after their arrival, mostly because I could use a break myself. For the past two weeks, I'd been tired, queasy and generally under the weather.

As I tap the top of the cardboard box with my fingers, I feel Mom's gaze fixed on me.

"Are you finally going to open them?" she asks.

"Are you done inspecting the kitchen?"

"For now," she says.

Sitting at the table, I wonder which box I should open first. A quick glance towards my mother doesn't provide any direction. She takes the seat across from me, serenely straight-faced, determined not to give anything away.

The box on my left is an old Christmas tin decorated with poinsettias. I recognize it from my youth. When I pick it up, I find it's heavier than I'd expected. Whatever's inside doesn't seem to have any room to move or rattle. It could be anything. Mom is the queen of repurposing and she's got entire closets full of stuff not stored in their original boxes to show for it. A pair of slide trays for a carousel projector, stacked inside a Stetson hatbox. Tarnished, mismatched silverware, crammed in an old makeup case. Fragile Christmas ornaments wrapped in tissue, stowed inside egg cartons.

Compared to the tin, the parcel to my right is feather-light and nondescript, made of thick white cardboard. Like its partner, nothing moves inside when I shake it. The top of the box has "TO:" and "FROM:" fields printed on it in bold black letters, so I assume it's a mailer. Is this simply a not-so-subtle hint that she wants more correspondence?

Mom lets out an impatient sigh.

I open it first.

Lifting the box's lid, I find a thin stack of paperwork laid on top of a large block of rigid foam. The papers are all marked with the official seal of the university where Dr. Lynch's laboratory is located. A bright blue booklet on the top of the pile is titled: *Living with HEREDITARY Colorectal Cancer.* Its table of contents includes such topics as: *Basic Genetics; Risks and Benefits of Genetic Testing;* and *Prevention Options.* The foam beneath the papers is partitioned into six sections, each containing a rubber-topped tube for collecting blood.

Mom says, "You said you wanted me to get you everything you'd need for the test, so here it is. Dr. Lynch's assistant said you can have the blood drawn here by anyone you like, so long as you ship it back to them right away. The instructions are all there, but you can always call the lab if you have any questions."

"All right," I say, putting the lid back on the box. "I'll get to it as soon as I can."

"I'll go with you to the doctor's office if you like," Mom offers.

"To give me a lollipop and hold my hand?"

"No." She shakes her head. "To answer any questions your doctor might have. Don't you think I know that you're not afraid of a little needle stick?"

I respect her persistence, but the test is the last thing I want either of us to think about while she's here. "Maybe I'll get it done next week," I concede, wanting to change the subject. "If there's time."

Sensing my discomfort, Mom changes her tack. "How about you open the other box? I think it might be just what you need."

Cradling the tin to my chest, I pry open the lid. There's a crumpled layer of wax paper hiding the tin's contents, but the scent gives it away. I breathe in the scents of ginger, clove, cinnamon and molasses. "Lebkuchen!" I say, fishing out one of the sugar-glazed cookies laden with dried fruits and nuts. From the first bite, my worries are quieted, my nervous stomach, settled.

Mom gives me a knowing look. "I made a double batch of dough last December and put half of it in the freezer. Something told me you might be needing it. Have you any news for me?"

I take another bite.

"Out with it, schnicklefritz. Don't keep me waiting."

How could she guess I was pregnant from over a thousand miles away? Shaking my head in disbelief, I say, "It was supposed to be a surprise."

Mom laughs and claps her hands. "I knew it! I heard it in your voice."

Of course she did. Suddenly weepy I say, "You always know exactly what I need."

I carry the test kit to the china cabinet at the other end of the kitchen and stow it inside. "Is it okay if I take a rain check on this? Just for the next few months."

Mom stands and gives me a warm hug. "So long as you don't forget it."

"I won't forget, Mom."

"Promise?"

"I promise."

We spend the next three weeks, Mom, Dad, Ian, the Kid and me, rock hounding at the beach, sitting around bonfires, playing board games, and eating too much lobster. I tell my parents repeatedly that it means the world to me to have them here and for them to see that the Kid and I are ridiculously happy.

"This place suits you," Mom says as she tugs a stray weed from between two rows of carrots in my vegetable garden. "You're beaming, your son's thriving, your marriage is solid and your family is growing. That makes leaving you a little easier on your dear mom and dad."

"I wish home wasn't so far away," I say.

"*This* is your home now, sweetie. This is where you belong."

The final morning of my parents' visit, I hustle around the kitchen with Mom, preparing food for them to eat during the first leg of their trip home. The radio is on while we work, tuned to *This Morning* on the CBC.

The host's voice echoes through the kitchen as we spread mustard and slap cold cuts onto slices of marble rye.

"Isn't that the woman who introduced *your* radio piece?" Mom asks.

"Yes," I answer. I'd written a first-person essay that'd been featured on the show, and had sent a cassette of it home to Mom and Dad after it aired. It was about a ninety-five-year-old woman I'd met in the grocery store who'd offered to teach me to box. "How many times did you listen to that piece?"

"Enough to know that you should keep writing. I sure hope you've been finding some time for it."

"A little, yes." Sharing my writing with others is a new experience for me. I'd been performing on stage since I was a child, but until that essay, my non-academic writing had been something I'd only done for myself. Having my work air on the radio had been a wonderful experience, but I wasn't sure if anything like it would ever happen again.

"So what are you working on?" Mom presses.

"Well, I took a workshop a while back with a CBC producer who specializes in radio documentaries. He loaned me some recording equipment so I can try my hand at interviewing people for a small project I've got in mind."

"What sort of people?"

"Women in the community, mostly."

"What do you talk to them about?"

"Local history and traditions. I found out that a midwife used to live in my house. The women used to come here to have their babies."

Mom gives my belly an affectionate pat. "And soon there'll be one more."

Early on a snowy morning in March, I wake to feel the first signs of labour. After I tell Ian, I call Mom.

"Is today the day?" she asks.

"It is."

Ian is pacing the floor beside me, waving his finger in circles in the air. He wants me to wrap it up.

"I'll have to call you back a little later, Mom. Ian needs to phone the midwife."

"Heavens, he hasn't called her yet?"

"I wanted to hear your voice first."

"Well, get some rest while you can, dear. I'll talk to you soon."

I call Mom several times throughout the day, between short walks and warm baths and labour pains. Each time we talk, I'm a little more distracted and breathless. Late afternoon I let her know that I won't be talking to her again until the baby is born.

She hadn't been too enthusiastic about my choosing to have a home birth, but in the end she'd said she was proud of me for weighing all the options and trusting my heart. Her trust in me had been the greatest gift of my life.

Just after sunset, a healthy baby boy slips from my body into the world. As a late winter storm rages outside, kicking up angry waves in the Bay, we are cradled within the walls of a house that's seen dozens of mothers give birth and hear their babies' first cries. "You are safe," I whisper to my new son. "You are loved."

Cuddled in bed with the baby, Ian and Eldest Son, I reach for the phone.

"I wish I could hold him," Mom says, tears in her voice. "I can't wait to meet him."

I can't help but feel that everything about this day—the joy, the wonder, the bliss—is because of her.

"I'll get home as soon as I can, Mom."

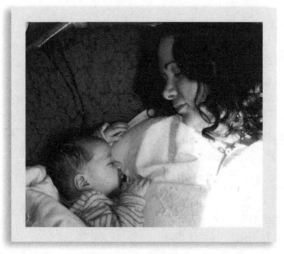

Holding Youngest Son, 2001

38.

Today's the Day

Eldest Son sends me a text while I'm in the car with Ian.

> **ES:** The lab called to say my results are in early. I have a phone call with a genetic counsellor today at 3:15. I'll call you afterwards!

> **AM:** Oh, wow. Dad and I are on our way into town, but we'll be home before then. I'll be waiting for your call. Love you!

I stare at my phone. I'd thought we were still a week away from this. Ian asks, "Everything all right?"

"He's getting his results today . . ."

"Should we turn around and head back home?"

"It won't be until this afternoon. We might as well get a few things done."

"Are you sure?"

At the moment, I'm not sure about anything.

"Yeah, I guess."

We carry on.

"How will I know what to do?" I ask Ian as we pull into the grocery store parking lot. I'm starting to panic. "How will I know what to say?"

"Just breathe," he says, turning off the car's engine.

"But what if I mess it up?"

He takes hold of my hand. "There isn't a wrong way."

I doubt that's true, but I don't voice the thought. I know he's being thoughtful and kind.

"You had a good mother," he says. "She taught you well. You won't mess this up."

All I can think is, *He'll never forget the words I say to him today.* "Do you think we should go to Halifax to be with him?"

Ian squeezes my hand. "Call him. You'll know more when you hear his voice."

I dial the number, take a deep breath.

"Hey—how's it going?" Eldest Son says.

"It goes," I reply. "You doing okay?"

"Sure," he says. "I'm ready."

He sounds strong, upbeat, so I don't press him further. Instead, I make an attempt at saying something I hope will give him comfort while he waits for the call. "No matter the result, it won't change who you are. You'll be exactly the same person you were when you woke up this morning, you'll just have learned something new about yourself."

It's far more complicated than that, but I'm trying not to say anything that could make it sound as if I've assumed the worst.

"Thanks, Mom," he says. "That helps a lot."

"Do you want me and Dad to come to Halifax?" I ask. "We could be there with you when you get the call."

"No, it's okay," he quickly responds. "How about I come home tomorrow, if that works for you?"

"Tomorrow's great."

Ian and I spend the morning grocery shopping, banking and eating lunch out, just as we'd planned. I'm there and not there, all at once. I keep asking Ian if I've done things right. Have I prepared Eldest Son for this moment? Have I explained things well enough to his younger brother? I don't want either of our boys to feel left in the dark.

There's no handbook for being a previvor, and I'm not sure it would matter if there was one. I keep thinking of how grateful I am to have had the parents I did, and that all my hoping, praying, and wishing that my sons' results will be negative won't make any difference.

Ian is valiantly patient as I flit between nervous chatter and bewildered silence.

"I thought we'd get more notice," I say as we leave our favourite lunch spot. "Now we're down to the wire . . . only a couple of hours away from *the* answer."

"It's probably better this way," Ian says, carefully, wisely, always with love. He hates it when I knot myself up with worry. Any time he can keep me from it, he does.

Normally we'd stop in at the local bookshop, or wander along the dykeland, but today I want to get home as soon as possible. As we pass by a crowded patio filled with laughter and sun-kissed faces, I think, *It's a perfect spring afternoon. Just like it was when I got my results from Dr. Lynch.* And it's exactly the same time of year, nearly to the day.

On our way home, we make a brief stop at our friends' house so Ian can drop off some beekeeping equipment for them. He'd helped them start a hive the previous spring and he's anxious to see how their bees have fared over the winter.

I'm pretty certain I won't be good company, so I wait in the car.

With the sunroof open, I hear the sound of honeybees buzzing overhead as they collect pollen from the catkins in the branches of a nearby willow. I love hearing them hard at work, doing everything in their power to make a go of it. We'd lost our three hives over the winter and won't be able to establish new ones until late June. The bees' absence in my life feels especially keen in this moment. My friend Holly comes to the side of the car and knocks on the window. "Hey, you," she says as I open the door.

"Hey, Holly," I say, getting out to hug her. "I've just been sitting here, listening to your bees. Sorry I didn't come inside, I figured you might be busy." She and her husband, Alan, are artists, and their work schedule is similar to mine and Ian's—some days are laid back, most are a race to the finish.

"I'm never too busy for you," she says with a smile.

She keeps me company as we wait for our husbands to wrap up their conversation. I don't mention Eldest Son or the call he'll soon be getting. She knows that I have Lynch syndrome, but not that my son is being tested for the gene. She and Alan have just become empty nesters, so any talk of our kids makes her sentimental and tender. I don't want to saddle her with this today.

Instead, I tell her that we'd lost our own hives over the winter. "Sometimes you do everything right and you still lose them. Ian says there wasn't anything else we could've done."

"I guess keeping bees can be like raising children," Holly says. "Sometimes they bring you joy, sometimes they break your heart."

3:00 P.M.

I put the groceries in the fridge, then sit at the kitchen table, the phone to my right, a box of tissues to my left. I know I'm going to cry one way or another—either from relief or guilt.

Although these last few minutes of yes-or-no before the news feel familiar, I find it far more difficult waiting for my son's results than I did my own. Clutching a tissue, I sit there.

4:20 P.M.

The phone rings.

I answer.

Eldest Son and I exchange hellos, then he cuts to the chase. "I tested positive for MSH2, Mom."

"Oh, sweetie," I say, eyes welling. "I'm so sorry." The guilt hits me first, followed by a crushing wave of sadness. I can hardly breathe.

"It's okay, Mom, honest."

My mind races to find the right words to fill the silence. My mother's voice fills the void first. *Snap out of it, Ami. He needs you.*

Wiping my eyes, I tell him, "I've thought about this moment a lot—what to do, what to say—and nothing I came up with was better than what your grandmother told me the day I got my results. She said, 'You've got a big job ahead, and it's not going to be easy, but I know you're up to the challenge because I know who you are.'"

"Thanks, Mom," he says. He sounds sombre, overwhelmed.

"I know I told you earlier that the results don't change who you are, but you should know that testing positive will likely change how you look at life. Some days it will be all you can and should think about, and other days it'll leave you feeling bold and full of big dreams because it's made you realize how foolish it is to wait around for 'someday.'"

"Yeah," he says, "that makes sense."

For the next few minutes, we talk over the information the lab sent him via email—recommended screenings and procedures; statistics and percentages relating to his cancer risk.

"Were you happy with how the lab conveyed things to you?" I ask.

"Actually, yes. They were really great. The genetic counsellor was friendly and clear. She walked me through everything step by step and answered all my questions."

"Was there anything that confused you or caught you off guard?"

"No. Not really."

"Good. The next step is to take your results to the genetics centre in Halifax. They'll be able to set you up with the specialists you need to see for your screenings."

I add, "Don't be surprised if you have to educate a few docs along the way. Not every GP knows about Lynch syndrome. It's our responsibility to keep medical practitioners informed. Read up on the latest research. Ask questions. Don't be quiet if you feel something's being missed. Your life depends on it."

I wonder if I'm laying too much on him all at once. But he needs to know about these things from the start. Part of me regrets not being there to say them in person, but I comfort myself with the fact that his girlfriend is there to give him support. "You've had a lot thrown at you in the last hour. Maybe you should get out in the sunshine and take a walk with your sweetheart."

"That sounds good. I think I will." Before he says goodbye, he says the words I was praying he wouldn't. "I'm sorry, Mom."

I can hardly bear it. "You have absolutely nothing to be sorry for."

"But I know it's not the result you wanted."

"It's not the one that anyone wants, but it's the one we both got and we'll get through this together. Right?"

"Right."

"Go have that walk and I'll see you tomorrow. If you need anything before then, just give me a call."

I motion to Ian, who's been listening in, to see if he wants to add something before we go.

He shakes his head, no.

"I love you, kiddo."

"I love you too, Mom."

The second I get off the phone, I take shelter in Ian's arms. Crying into his chest I sob, "Why couldn't it end with me?"

That night, I wrote a letter to my mother.

May 7, 2018

Dear Mom,

I'm sorry.

The day I got my results and told you the news, I made a terrible mistake.

You, feeling my pain and yours, started to cry, and I told you not to. (As if you had a choice.)

Still fighting my way through what I'd just learned, I wanted to comfort you, to stop you from feeling (sadness, despair, guilt) because I love you.

And because I didn't understand the importance of letting you in, to share in a moment where everything changed, for me, for you, for us.

I'm sorry.

I had no right.

I stole something precious that I can never make right.

Maybe if I'd been with you, looked into your eyes, witnessed your tears, felt the familiar gesture of your hand on mine, where you'd placed it so many times—to hold me back from danger, or myself—maybe then I would've let you cry until you were sure that everything would be fine.

Or fine enough, for now.

But I didn't know how it felt, until now.

Today I learned what it is to be a mother who discovers that her child must now face challenges, hardships and sorrow, because of her.

It is and isn't my fault. Just like it was and wasn't yours.

I understand.

And I'm sorry.

Can you see them? My boys?

If you can, then you already know that they possess gifts that came from you; grown from seeds you planted in their hearts during moments that were all too brief.

They are quick to laugh. Eager to embrace joy.

They are champions of fairness and truth.

They love music and beauty, and questioning the world around them, not with cynicism, but with generosity of spirit.

They are more confident than I am.

And less hesitant, which is good.

They are twinned souls who will carry each other for the rest of their lives—past my lifetime, God willing, as it should be.

Because of you, I know that all is not lost.

Because of you, I revere honesty and patience and kindness.

Because of you, I believe that magic can occur at any turn, confronting me with tenderness, beauty and wonder—when I least expect it, when I need it most.

Thank you for teaching me what it means to be loved, and that no love is ever wasted.

Although you are not here, you are with me still.

I love you to the moon and back.

Ami

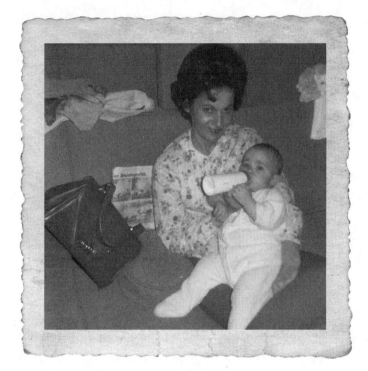

Mom and me, 1968

39.

Homecoming

Michigan and Indiana, September 11, 2001, morning
Ian, Eldest Son, the baby and I are at Lori's house in Michigan. As
I rush back and forth between the kitchen and the bathroom to help
with the breakfast dishes and get the kids ready for the day, a terrible
image on the living room TV catches my eye. The television screen
takes up half the wall, so the sight of billowing clouds of smoke
streaming from one of the World Trade Center towers looks like a
trailer for a new action film. I cry out when I realize it's not.

Ian is standing next to me when the second plane hits.

"This can't be real," I whisper. "How could this happen?"

The announcer keeps talking about how clear and blue the skies
were earlier in the morning. She uses phrases like, *possible accident, still
unconfirmed, waiting for word.*

Ian shakes his head. "I don't think it was an accident."

We'd left Nova Scotia the week before, on a road trip we'd dubbed
"the 2001 Baby McKay World Tour." After stopping in Ontario to
visit Ian's grandmother, we'd crossed the border en route to my parents' place. My sister's house had been the perfect overnight stop
before travelling on to Indiana.

Our mini-van was loaded with all the things that two adults, an
eight-year-old and a six-month-old would need for a month-long trip:
sippy cups, juice boxes, graham crackers, pretzels, baby food, pacifiers, a

charged-up Game Boy and dozens of assorted CDs—Raffi, the Muppets, Peter, Paul and Mary. I'd also filled a backpack with notebooks, pens and a small kit of recording gear on loan from the CBC.

The interviews I'd previously taped with the women of my community had eventually become part of a radio documentary about the history of midwifery. After it had aired, the producer I'd worked with, Dick Miller, asked if I'd like to team up with him again. When I'd said it would have to wait until I got back from a family vacation, he'd asked, "Where're you headed?"

"Ontario, Michigan and Indiana, to show off the baby."

"Got any interesting plans for while you're there? Anything out of the ordinary?" He was always angling for a good story.

"Actually, yes," I'd answered. "My mom wants me to have my blood drawn for a genetic test to see if I'm at risk for certain kinds of cancer."

"Wow," he'd said. "Sounds heavy. Are you going to do it?"

"I think so . . . maybe." I hadn't forgotten my promise to my mother, but I wasn't sure if a vacation was the right time for me to get the test.

"So you haven't made up your mind?"

"Not yet."

"Hmm," he says, scribbling on a pad of paper. "Tell me more about that."

By the end of our conversation, I'd brought Dick up to speed on the ins and outs of Lynch syndrome, and he'd fetched me a canvas bag with a reporter's field kit.

"Only do what feels comfortable," he'd said. "You don't have to document anything that feels too personal or invasive."

"Thanks," I'd said, as I got up to leave. "Maybe it'll help me make sense of things."

Between truck stops, road construction delays, and countless rounds of twenty questions, I'd written a long list of questions of my own.

Some were for my relatives who'd already had cancer:

Can you describe your symptoms?

Did you think it was cancer from the start?

What did your doctor think it was?

What do you think of the genetic test?

Do you think that being positive for the gene would've made any difference in your diagnosis and treatment?

What do you say to those in the family who don't wish to be tested?

Others were for those who hadn't:

Are you aware of our family's history of cancer?

Have you shared it with your doctor?

How do you feel about the test?

Do you worry when you have stomach pain or intestinal trouble?

Are you scared of getting cancer?

The more questions I wrote for my family, the more I had for myself.

Do I really want to know if I have the gene?

If I test positive, how will I feel?

Will I waste the rest of my life worrying about test results and prophylactic surgeries?

How many associated cancers are there?

Should I have a hysterectomy?

Should I not have any more children?

Everything about cancer terrified me. If it could get to my mom, it could surely get to me.

September 11, 2001, afternoon

Every airport in the US has been shut down. Federal buildings evacuated. Schools are in lockdown mode. The military is on high alert.

Shortly after we get to my parents' house, Brian calls from the army base in South Carolina to say that they're on lockdown too, so he won't be able to travel to see his son this weekend as planned. He has no idea how long things will have to stay this way. I have no idea what to tell my son.

People in New York are searching for the missing. Some have gone so far as to pin photos of friends and family to their clothing in hopes that someone might recognize their loved ones as they walk the streets. It's a desperate, heartbreaking act, but I understand their desire to do something, anything.

Over dinner, my parents speak of their childhoods during the Second World War. It's surreal to hear them sift through their memories as the TV flickers with images of smouldering rubble and debris. Mom lived in a town with a gun factory at one end and a bomber assembly plant at the other. "Every night I'd fall asleep to the sound of gunshots and planes flying overhead. I knew things were much worse overseas, but that only made me more fearful that eventually we'd be invaded."

"Everything went to the war effort back then," Dad says. "We went without essentials, like gas and food, for long stretches at a time. Your grandpa used to take steam belts from old farm equipment to make new soles for my shoes. I don't know if people know how to pull together like that anymore."

Mom closes her eyes. "Today was scarier than anything I've ever experienced in my life."

As I listen to them, my fears about the test seem trivial. All I can think is, *No amount of fear can ever make us safe.*

Sunday, September 16, 2001
As the world carries on as best it can, Mom throws an impromptu family reunion. Between stirring baked beans and making hamburger patties she says, "It'll be good for us to get together. Family is important, especially in times like these."

By noon, the backyard is full of siblings, cousins, aunts, uncles, nieces and nephews. No one has any concrete answers about the state of the world, but everyone is eager to talk about it.

I set up my recording equipment in my parents' bedroom at the back of the house, thinking we might as well talk about cancer while we've got mortality on our minds. With my baby in my arms, I wind my way through croquet matches and past the picnic table, quietly issuing invitations to family members to have a chat with me about Lynch syndrome. I have no idea if I'll have any takers, but at least it gives me something to do.

My uncle Jamie's middle daughter, my cousin Holly, jumps in first. She'd tested positive back in June and gotten a hysterectomy shortly thereafter. She's thirty-seven.

Of her five siblings, one has also tested positive; another, negative. Her three other siblings still refuse to take the test.

After handing the baby off to Ian, I lead Holly to my makeshift studio. Memories of family picnics past flash through my mind. Holly and I used to love eavesdropping on our older sisters as they talked about music, clothes and boys.

I press record, and ask, "Did you have to think about having the test done, or was it 'Yes' from the start?"

"Instantly I was gonna do it," she says. "I felt like I probably did have the gene, so I figured the benefits outweighed anything else. I also felt that I owed it to my daughter. I wanted to know whether or not there was a chance I'd passed the gene on to her."

Her confidence floors me. There's no second-guessing or fear. She reminds me of my mother.

"When they showed us the family tree," she says, "when I saw who'd previously had cancer, I just couldn't imagine not having the test done. It's a huge time bomb, ticking away. I don't understand people not doing it. For me the fear of the unknown was far worse than knowing."

My brother Doug also agrees to a chat. This comes as a surprise to me because he and my eldest brother are both still resisting Mom's campaign to take the test. He's already had thyroid cancer, though it wasn't attributed to Lynch syndrome. Even though he's pretty sure he's positive, there's no way he'll know for certain unless he gets tested.

"There's no guarantee that the results will remain private," he says. "I just don't think I should take the risk." Turning the tables on me he asks, "How do you feel about it?"

"I'm nervous," I admit. "But I'm trying to put on a brave face in front of Mom."

"Why would you do that?" he asks. "Are you that worried about the results?"

"Kind of, yes. I keep thinking that if I test positive, Mom will feel guilty about it."

He frowns. "You think so? She has no control over that."

"You're right," I say. "But I can't imagine how I'd feel if I found out one of my children had the gene. I think if I have it, I won't have any more kids."

"Really?"

"They say that women who carry the gene should have a hysterectomy once they're done having children, to eliminate the risk of certain cancers."

"And are you done having kids?"

"It's one thing to find out you're positive after you've completed your family, but it's quite another to pass the gene on to a child after knowing you're positive . . . I just don't think I could handle it."

Doug's knee begins to bounce. "Mom had colon cancer and she's still here. I've had cancer and I'm still kicking. I wouldn't let it scare you off too bad."

"But it's not like catching a cold, Doug. You know as well as anybody, you can't just shake cancer off."

"The sooner they detect it, the sooner they can get to it."

I'm starting to think Mom has put him up to this. "You sure don't sound like someone who doesn't want to get tested."

After a long pause he asks, "Do you ever worry that if we don't participate in the study, we might be missing the big picture?"

"I'm not sure what you mean."

"Sometimes I think this thing is bigger than us and our insecurities. I don't want to shortchange the folks that are doing the research in any way. Their focus isn't on whether or not you have more kids or the state of my health insurance. Their focus is on the big picture, on how cancer works and how to help others. Maybe we should think about that."

I think of our mother's devotion to Dr. Lynch's work and the faith she has in his team. She doesn't give that sort of trust freely or easily to anyone. It has to be earned. She's never asked me to do anything she wouldn't be willing to do herself, never put me in a situation that has caused me to doubt her. Waiting for her children to do the right thing must be breaking her heart.

"You're right," I say, finding some clarity at last. "I'm going to get my blood drawn as soon as I can and worry about the rest later. If you can find a way that makes sense for you to take it, then I think you should too." (And he will, the following year.)

Tuesday, September 17, 2001

One week after the attacks, Mom drives me to the hospital to get the test. It's the same hospital where I was born.

As we travel along the streets of my hometown, I notice every house has an American flag prominently displayed on its porch or front lawn. It reminds me of when the town puts on its finery for Independence Day, only today the streets are quiet, the sidewalks nearly empty. For all the talk that's been going around the last few days about patriotism and national unity, people have, by and large, stayed inside, glued to their television and computer screens. The general attitude, at least in this part of the country, isn't one of resilience, but fear.

Mom seizes the opportunity to touch on mine while she's got me captive in the car. Turning the radio off, she turns to pushing my buttons instead. "The other night we were talking about whether or not you were going to have any more kids, and you said that if you tested positive, that would be reason enough for you not to have any more children."

She is absolutely relentless.

"Well," she goes on, "I've been thinking about it a lot, and I have to say I'm really not happy with that."

"Mom," I say, wishing she hadn't chosen to discuss this now. "I've got two amazing kids, I'm thirty-three years old, and I'm not sure I want to have any more children anyway."

"Exactly," she says. "You're not sure."

"Mom, please . . ." She'd had a hysterectomy when I was five, due to fibroids and excessive monthly bleeding. She was forty. She and Dad already had the family they'd always wanted, so the choice had been an easy one to make. The spectre of the endometrial cancers her cousin, aunt and grandmother had suffered from had only provided added incentive. *Is my position so different?* I bite my tongue and resist the urge to argue.

"Hear me out on this," she insists. "I don't want the results of this test to dictate that part of your life. It's not like these cancers can't be treated. Having the gene isn't a death sentence. The ability for you to know whether you have it or not is a gift. Think of the strength and courage our ancestors had to have in the face of difficult times. I've called on that courage countless times to help me survive instead of allowing despair to take me over. I'll be damned if I'll let it take you."

My brother had been right—this wasn't about our fears and worries. It was about being wildly, passionately, outrageously devoted to life. "It won't, Mom. I promise."

"Good," she says, pulling into the hospital parking lot. "Now go in there and let the nurse take your blood."

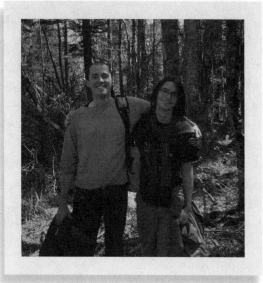

40.

Into the Woods

Scots Bay, Nova Scotia, May 13, 2018

Eldest Son comes home bearing gifts—a homemade Key lime pie and a large manila folder. It's his second visit since receiving his results. "Happy Mother's Day!" he says as he sets the folder and the pie on the kitchen island.

I give him a hug. Picking up the folder, I ask, "What's this?"

"Copies of my paperwork from the genetic counsellor."

"For me?"

He nods. "For the historical record."

We'd talked a lot since he'd gotten his results, discussing everything from the state of his emotions to the long list of to-dos that comes with Lynch syndrome. The day after he found out he was positive, he'd sent his results to both our family doctor and the genetics centre in Halifax. He'd also sent me a photo of one of the walls in his painting studio, covered with notes and pages from his sketchbook, tacked up in a long timeline. *Plans for the future,* he'd written. *Big dreams.*

"I'll be sure to take good care of this," I say, then swipe the edge of the pie with my finger and stick it in my mouth.

"Mom!"

"But it's Mother's Day."

My only wish for the day is that all four of us go for a hike in the woods, like we've done for the past several years running, our own Mother's Day rite of spring.

Today, the weather is perfect—clear skies with a cool breeze off the Bay. Blessedly, there are no blackflies yet.

As we make our way to the forest through a scrubby patch of alders, red-winged blackbirds and tree swallows swoop and chatter. The boys have spent the last few years making gentle trails through the woods behind the house, treading lightly on the land so as not to disturb the animals that call this place home.

Just as we enter a mossy grove of spruce, a pair of ravens perch on top of an old hemlock and begin to squawk and jeer at a red-tailed hawk that's circling overhead. While they stand guard over their roost, I sit on a fallen tree that stretches across a small, rushing stream. This is the place where my mother has often appeared to me in my dreams, sitting on this same log, placidly smiling as she dangles her feet over the water.

"Should we go this way?" Youngest Son asks, pointing in the direction of a narrow, rugged trail that winds up a steep hill.

His simple question weighs more than it should. I feel instantly sentimental, helplessly maternal. He'd spent the better part of the morning talking with his brother about where he might like to attend university, which had felt far too soon for me.

"Sure," I say, giving myself a mental kick. The path he's chosen leads to a meadow that sits atop a ridge that overlooks the sea. That'll be our reward for the climb.

The trail is rougher than usual, littered with tree roots and windfall and patches of leaves matted and slick from spring rains, but when we arrive at the hill's crest, we're met with a great stretch of sparsely treed land carpeted with spring beauties.

Among the tiny pink and white flowers are fiddleheads, Dutchman's breeches and red trilliums pushing their way through winter's debris, plants whose names my mother taught me. Reaching the trail's end, we scatter along the ridge to stare out at the sea below. We're alone up here, away from roads and buildings and homes and all the sounds that buzz through our daily lives. There are no signs that anyone else has been here for some time, except for the occasional faded blue dot of spray paint on a tree trunk, left by a wayward trail-blazer. Stopping to take it all in, I listen to my sons nearby, talking about an upcoming camping trip.

Youngest Son wants their excursion to count towards the "Adventurous Journey" portion of his silver Duke of Edinburgh Award, so he's in charge of every aspect of the trip—food, camping gear, trail maps, the first aid kit. Eldest Son is more than willing to be his little brother's enthusiastic sidekick. Turning my face to the sun, I close my eyes and hope that Ian and I have given them all that they need to navigate life.

You're not done yet, my mother's voice whispers.

My mother had chosen to lead me by example rather than by the nose. Maybe it was because I was her youngest or, more likely, because of my stubborn nature, but more often than not, she'd taught me life's lessons through actions not lectures.

Even when cancer came knocking for the second time in her life, she'd never treated it as a "fight," because she'd felt there was nothing to be gained by believing that she was in a battle that could either be won or lost. She'd chosen to let go of her anger and show the disease a strange sort of respect—so it wouldn't weigh her heart down and consume her spirit.

After it was removed, she'd even insisted on keeping the port from her chemotherapy—a hard knob of plastic similar in size and shape to a champagne cork that had been embedded in her chest to deliver her medication—over the objections of the doctor who said she couldn't have it. Mom always had a way of talking people out of shouldn'ts, and into the impossible.

She kept the port in a little bottle on the vanity next to her bed. After living inside my mother for nearly a year, her flesh had begun to claim it, and it hadn't made a clean exit from her body. Feathery strands of tissue, ghostly white, still clung to it as it bobbed in a tiny sea of formaldehyde.

When she showed it to me she'd said, "I stare at it sometimes to remind myself that a person can die while they're still alive, simply by not choosing to live."

It's taken me a long time to understand what she'd meant by that.

Worry can be pernicious. Left unchecked, it slowly bleeds the soul of joy and replaces it with fear.

There's no room for "why me?" with Lynch syndrome. The mutation is only part, not all of who I am. Rather than let it rule me, I choose to fold the rituals of annual screenings and tests into the cycles and rhythms of my life. If I give the disease the space and attention it needs (no more, no less), just as my mother did, then I'll give myself space for everything else—hope, love, dreams, bliss.

Of the paths ahead to travel, some will have twists and turns and steep climbs. But if I look at each day as my mother did, as an invitation to live, then I think I'll be all right.

"Ready to go?" Youngest Son asks, eager to tackle a different trail on the way home.

Smiling, I say, "Lead the way."

41

What Dreams May Come

Scots Bay, Nova Scotia, April 8, 2002

It's been two hundred days since I had my blood drawn. At some point during every one of them, I've thought about what my results will be. I have no idea when they'll come.

I believe that I'm positive. I'll be shocked if I'm not.

I've been having nightmares on and off for weeks.

Once, I dreamed that Dr. Lynch's lab called and said they needed more of my blood, "just to be sure." This time they required twenty-eight cups of it, rather than six small tubes—four cups more than the average human body holds. Halfway through filling cup number fourteen, the nurse stopped and told me that she'd made a mistake. "You'll have to come back tomorrow and start all over again."

Last night I dreamed that I went to the dentist to get a cavity filled. They knocked me out so I couldn't feel anything, couldn't move, but I could still see all that was happening. To my horror, the dentist took out a scalpel and slit my belly, "to see what's inside," she said. Then she pulled out my intestines and several other organs because they were, in her words, "no good." I watched helplessly as she shoved crumpled garbage bags into my empty gut then sewed me shut.

My youngest son, my baby, is now a year old. He's walking on his own, discovering the world around him, becoming aware of everything.

How old was I when I first became aware of cancer?

I remember, as early as kindergarten, feeling so confused and worried by the word that whenever someone said it, I got a bellyache.

Sometimes I'd even throw up. Not so different than I'm feeling now. I'm paralyzed by the thought of getting cancer. I don't want to be sick like that. I know it can be treated, even cured, but I don't want to go through the pain and torture of it.

I've started keeping an audio diary to help make sense of things. It's been good (so far) to sit with my thoughts every night and confess them into quiet nothingness.

Dick Miller, the CBC Radio producer who suggested I record my journey with genetic testing, says I can change my mind at any time about the documentary, scrap the whole thing if I want. My inclination (at least for today) is to go ahead with it. Dr. Lynch has agreed to let me interview him on the day he gives me my results. His assistant said I'd have an answer in fourteen weeks. It's been thirty.

Should I call the lab and ask why it's taking so long?

Just after lunch the phone rings.

"Ami?" A woman's voice says. "It's Patty."

I can count on one hand the times I've spoken to my ex's wife on the phone.

"Hi, Patty," I say. "Everything okay?"

"No," she answers, her voice trembling. "Brian's dead."

My legs go weak. "Oh, God. What happened?"

She cries as she recites a list of details that make no sense. "They found his truck at the park by the river. They found his body on the trail."

It must've been an accident, I think. Brian was an avid cyclist who had a bad habit of listening to music while he biked. How many times had I warned him not to do that?

"A woman spotted him while she was out walking with her baby in a stroller. He was just lying there, in his uniform."

"In his uniform?" *Was it a brain aneurysm? A mugging gone bad?*

"It was suicide," she says. "He shot himself in the head."

"Shit," I say, shocked. "Do you have someone with you? Are you going to be all right?" Patty's family, like mine, was back in Indiana. I wasn't sure if she had anyone to lean on in South Carolina.

"He left a note," she says.

"For you?" I ask. I can't bear the thought of it being for my son. *How am I ever going to explain this to him?*

"Yes," she answers. "It was in the truck."

She doesn't tell me what it says and I don't ask.

As soon as I hang up, I look at the clock. In less than two hours my son will get off the school bus and walk through the door.

I slump to the floor and cry.

Ian finds me after he's put the baby down for a nap.

"Brian's gone," I sob, unable to think. "He's dead."

"What? How?" He sits next to me and takes hold of my hand.

One by one, I stutter through the things Patty said. The more I think of what Brian has done, the more confused and angry I become—with him, with the world, with myself. "Why didn't I see this coming?"

The last conversation I'd had with him had been just after Christmas. He'd told me that he wasn't happy in the army, that things hadn't turned out the way he'd hoped.

"Can't you quit?" I'd asked. "Just not re-up next time around?"

"Patty wants to have a baby. I need to have a secure job if we decide to have a kid."

"You'll figure something out. That's great news by the way, that Patty's trying to get pregnant."

"Is it?" he'd asked.

"Sure. Why wouldn't it be?"

"Because I'm a crap dad."

I hadn't been sure what to say to that.

"I sucked from the start and I haven't gotten any better over the years. I barely know our kid anymore. I didn't even call him on Christmas. I'd never see him at all if it wasn't for you making the arrangements and my dad buying the plane tickets."

He hadn't been wrong about any of it, but it'd seemed petty to call him out on it when he was feeling so low. "Only you and Patty know what's best for your relationship. And as far as your relationship with our son goes, it's never too late to try to make things better."

"He's got a good father now," Brian countered. "He doesn't need me."

"Ian's a great dad but that doesn't mean the Kid no longer needs you in his life. He loves you. You know that."

Brian made a hasty retreat. "I gotta go."

"Don't you want to at least say hi to him?"

"Not tonight."

"All right," I'd said, biting my tongue. "I'll just tell him his daddy Brian says hi."

After a long pause, Brian said, "He doesn't have to call me Dad anymore."

"That's bullshit, Brian, and you know it."

He'd hung up.

Pacing the kitchen floor, I ask Ian, over and over again, "What am I going to say to him?" I spiral into a crying jag.

"What can I do for you?" Ian calmly asks. "What do you need?"

"I need my mom." I whimper. "I want my mother."

Ian picks up the phone and dials my parents' number. He breaks the news, then hands me the phone.

"Oh, sweetie," Mom says. "I'm so sorry."

The sound of her voice brings on more tears. "I don't think I can do this, Mom."

"Don't talk," she says. "Just listen."

For the next twenty minutes she repeatedly tells me she loves me and that I'm made of "strong stuff."

I hear my father in the background quietly adding his support, and feel the warmth of my husband's hand on my shoulder as my mother works to bring me back to my senses and myself.

"You're going to be fine," she says before we say goodbye. "And so will our boy."

Within the hour, Brian's father, Bill, calls and attempts to orchestrate next steps, putting things in order as a way of combating grief. "I'll be helping Patty with the funeral," he says.

"That's good."

"Just let me know how many plane tickets you'll need and I'll make all the arrangements."

"I can't think about that now," I say. "I need to figure out what to tell my son."

"Tell him it was an accident. Tell him Brian was riding his bike. For God's sake, Ami, the boy's only eight years old. He doesn't need to know."

I know Bill means well. I know he loves his grandson. But his advice doesn't sit right with me. "I've never lied to my son, and I'm not about to start now."

Just before the Kid's bus is set to come rumbling down the road, a representative from the US Army calls to say he'll be flying to Nova Scotia in a few weeks to discuss the details of Brian's passing with me.

"I'm not Brian's wife," I say. "Why me?"

"You're the legal guardian to his child."

"What's there to discuss?"

"The conclusions of the investigation, ma'am."

"The investigation?"

"Into the matter of his death. It's protocol, ma'am."

"Will my son need to be present?"

"No, ma'am."

"Good."

I can hear the sound of papers shuffling. He's clearly talking from a script. "I must also inform you that an officer from the RCMP will be visiting your place of residence within the next forty-eight hours."

"Why?" I ask.

"To deliver the US Army's condolences to you and your son."

"That's not necessary."

"It's protocol, ma'am," he repeats.

I think of the tiny village where we live and the handful of houses that dot the dirt road that leads to our house. Police cars never come out this way unless something's terribly wrong. My neighbour calls me in a panic whenever she sees I've left my laundry on the line in the rain. I'll need to find a way to break the news to her before the officer shows up. "Could they at least call first?"

"I'll look into that, ma'am."

The Kid is full of excitement when he gets home. Racing through the back door, he takes off his coat and shoes, then unzips his backpack and pours its contents on the living room couch. Pushing aside Fruit Roll-up wrappers and Pokémon cards, he grabs a spiral-bound notebook and proudly opens it to a page that bears a primitive drawing of a planet in shades of blue, green, grey and black. Below the picture is a caption, written in jagged but considered eight-year-old script: *The Dark World.*

"I started writing a story," he proudly declares. "It's about another planet where there's magic and dragons and castles. I'm illustrating it myself."

"It looks awesome, kiddo," I say, wishing we could fly to his imaginary world right this minute. A silence falls as he looks into my face. "Have you been crying, Mom?" he asks, staring up at me with big eyes. "It looks like you've had tears."

"I have, sweetie. Something very sad happened today."

Aside from a pet goldfish that'd gone belly-up after the move from Chicago, he's never experienced death.

"What is it?" he asks, lip already quivering.

I can hear Ian upstairs, checking on the baby who's now awake.

"Your daddy Brian died this morning," I slowly say. The words feel too blunt but I can't take them back now.

After staring at me for a silent second, my son asks, "Was he sick?"

"Yes. He was."

"Couldn't the doctors fix it?"

"They didn't get the chance."

I've made sure that my answers aren't lies, but doorways to the truth. We'll pass through them together in the coming hours and days.

My son clings to me, buries his head against my chest as he lets out an anguished wail.

"I love you," I say, holding him close. Nothing else matters for now.

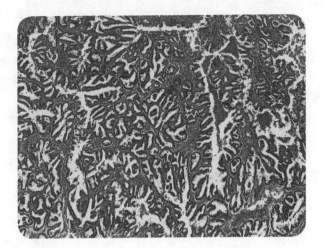

42.

Ruffles and Lace

Scots Bay, Nova Scotia, June 15, 2018

As the sun sets over the Bay, the evening sky is awash with brilliant strokes of red, pink, violet and blue. This particular kind of near-summer light has been considered a sign of hope in this tiny community for centuries. *Red sky at night, sailor's delight.* Tomorrow will be smooth sailing.

Turning from my studio window to my computer, I focus on one last bit of work for the day, a meditation on an image that's come to me across the miles and through the ether: a digitized slide of a tissue sample from Pauline's cancer. A pathologic ghost.

It, too, is made up of reds, pinks, violets and blues. It, too, is in my view at a moment of transition—from day to night, spring to summer, one month shy of the ninety-ninth anniversary of Pauline's death.

A few days after that milestone, I'll celebrate my fiftieth birthday, and this year-long expedition into the inner depths of my existence will come to an end.

The cellular portrait of Pauline's cancer is part of a collection that the University of Michigan's Pathology Department has painstakingly created for me from Family G tissue blocks they retrieved from their archives. The process involved several steps, each requiring steady hands and a meticulous eye for detail. Razor-thin ribbons of tissue from cancerous tumours had to be extracted from the decades-old paraffin blocks, then sliced, cleaned, set and stained before they could be magnified for digitization. They've sent twenty-two images in total, eight from Pauline's endometrial cancer in 1919; seven from my great-grandmother Tillie's first cancer in 1931; and seven from her second in 1933. All of them were made when the sisters' lives were hanging in the balance between life and death.

To Aldred Warthin and his successor, Carl Weller, the original samples, taken by their own hands, had served as physical evidence of the theory they'd so desperately wished to prove.

Of Pauline's tissues, Warthin had written: *Haemorrhage from the uterus developed suddenly without other symptoms; a diagnostic curettage showed advanced adenocarcinoma of the endometrium. Hysterectomy was performed in less than a week, and the uterus showed complete adenocarcinomatous infiltration of the entire wall body of the uterus, involving the bladder and broad ligament. The patient died of peritonitis within a few days.*

Of Tillie's, Weller had noted: *Atrophic ovaries with hyaline corpora fibrous. Leiomyoma in uterine wall. Chronic fibroid salpingitis. Recent partial curettage. Area of recent adenocarcinoma in endometrium, but no deep invasion of myometrium in the area examined. . . . The prognosis should still be good. Cystic cervical glands.*

To me, the image of Pauline's cancer symbolizes hope, even though I know I'm looking at deadly chaos, nature gone awry.

I'd seen images of her cancer before today, but they'd been grainy, black-and-white figures scanned from a blurry photocopy of an article in an old medical journal that'd been gathering dust on Dr. Lynch's shelf. Looking at them had been like peering through old windows streaked and mottled with dirt. Still, they'd been the only portraits of my great-great-aunt I'd ever seen.

Today's images are in fresh, saturated hues that are shocking to my eyes. The details are so clear, I can zoom in like a satellite moving its gaze from the outer reaches of space to a single glistening raindrop perched on the tip of a blade of grass. Every whorl, spot, curve and swirl of the disease is crisp and clear.

Staring at the canyons and tributaries of Pauline's fate, it occurs to me that I should probably find someone who knows the finer points of histology to sit with me and translate the image into language I can understand. *Not yet*, I think. For now, I'm content to gaze at it in wonder.

What strikes me most about it are its delicate intricacies—the deeper I go inside the image, the more I'm reminded of the shirred ruffles and dotted tulle, French knots and Swiss lace of Pauline's dressmaking.

Placing an image of Tillie's first cancer next to Pauline's, I look at them side by side, orchestrating a moment between the two sisters that they never shared in real life. Their endometrial cancers occurred over a decade apart, and yet they contain similar features, just as the living sisters had.

Is it wrong for me to feel such attachment to these slices of illness, disease and death? Am I manufacturing meaning that isn't there? This is the same question I ask myself every time I sit down to write.

I once asked Dr. Stern, the internist who'd performed all my colonoscopies, how he managed to identify cancers during a scope.

Comparing it to identifying birds, he'd said, "It's a balance of probabilities. If I see a Baltimore oriole in the backyard, then within point one of a second I know what it is. And I know what it isn't. But if I see an alder flycatcher but don't hear it calling, I have to take further steps to identify it: take a photograph and analyze the ratio of the tail to the body and so forth. Some of it is pattern recognition, some of it is actual measurements, and some of it is experience."

If you want to identify something properly, you have to be willing to see it in different ways.

I've spent the better part of a year examining my fate through the lenses of science, story, history, memory and being. The big picture is no less complicated than it was when I started, but it is clearer. Every observation I've made while sorting through the past has led to understanding, discovery and meaning.

If you want to properly tell a story, you have to be willing to write it a thousand ways.

And then you must be brave enough to share it with others.

O me! O life! of the questions of these recurring,
Of the endless trains of the faithless, of cities fill'd with the foolish,
Of myself forever reproaching myself, (for who more foolish than I,
*   and who more faithless?)*
Of eyes that vainly crave the light, of the objects mean, of the struggle
*   ever renew'd,*
Of the poor results of all, of the plodding and sordid crowds I see around me,
Of the empty and useless years of the rest, with the rest me intertwined,
The question, O me! So sad, recurring—What good amid these, O me, O life?

Answer.
That you are here—that life exists and identity,
That the powerful play goes on, and you may contribute a verse.
—Walt Whitman

43.

Daughter of Family G

Halifax, Nova Scotia, May 13, 2002

On a sunny afternoon in mid-May, I put on a pair of headphones and sit in front of a microphone at the CBC Radio studios in Halifax. It's not the typical way a person receives the results of a genetic test, but I've decided that it's my way.

As I sit alone in the recording booth with just a notebook and a cup of water by my side, my producer, Dick Miller, is behind a wall of soundproof glass, manning the controls. I haven't felt this nervous in, well, maybe ever. "I've booked the studio for an hour and half," he says, his voice steady in my headphones. "We've got plenty of time for everything you need to do."

After a quick review of my notes, I look at a clock that's fixed high on the studio wall: 12:02.

"Let me know when you're ready to call the lab," Dick says.

Giving him a thumbs-up, I say, "Ready."

First I speak with Dr. Lynch's assistant, Ali. She's in charge of walking me through an interview that will be used as part of Creighton's Hereditary Cancer Research Center's continuing study on Family G.

Some of the questions are straightforward and easily answered, but others are more difficult to hear, let alone consider. Even though I know they're coming, they still make me wince.

"Do you think that you're positive or negative for the marker?" Ali asks.

"Positive."

"If you find out you're positive, will you have a hysterectomy?"

"Probably, eventually, yes." I still haven't come to terms with that. She says if I have the gene, I should strongly consider having my uterus and ovaries removed, maybe even my colon. She reminds me that if I test positive, I may have already passed it on to my children. After we finish the survey, she connects me to Dr. Lynch so I can interview him before he gives me my results. It's my turn to ask the questions. They've been written in my notebook for months.

1. How did your research into Family G begin?

2. What are the main differences between someone who has the genetic marker and someone who doesn't?

3. What are the benefits to having genetic testing done?

4. What have been the biggest breakthroughs in recent years?

His answers are precise and clear, exactly as I expected. I already know much of what he's got to say about the syndrome and his work, but it's good to have a verbal account of it all, in his voice.

"The discovery of the mismatch repair germline mutations played an extremely important role in hereditary cancer research. Their implementation in testing individuals who are presumed to be at high Lynch syndrome risk has been the high point of my career. It's what finally made clinical diagnosis legitimate. And for that, I have you and your family to thank, for helping us all these years."

With each response he brings us closer to the moment of truth, until I eventually say, "I guess that's all the questions I have for now. I suppose we should get down to the nitty-gritty."

"Yep," he says. "Okay."

His voice cracks and falters as he delivers the news. "I really feel badly telling you this but you *did* inherit the gene. You *do* have the mutation."

Oh God, I think, *I'm positive.*

Last night I'd allowed myself five minutes to fantasize that I was negative. That will never happen again.

Once Dr. Lynch hangs up, Ali comes back on the line. "Ami?" she says. "I'm so sorry."

"Oh, Ali, it's okay." I'm trying (and failing) not to cry.

"I feel bad for you. I can sense tears because I've got tears in my eyes too."

"I thought I was ready to hear it, but maybe it's always shocking to find out you're positive, no matter how much you prepare for it."

"It is," she says. "It truly is. But like Dr. Lynch stated, the positive thing about this is that you're in total control of your healthcare."

I've never felt more powerless in my life.

Looking up from my notebook, I catch sight of Dick through the glass. He's wiping away tears.

When he comes to my side of the studio to check in and regroup, he asks, "You doing all right?"

I take a sip of water and blow my nose. "I won't lie, that was pretty rough."

"I know we were going to tape you calling your mom next, but if you want to go home and do that in private, I'll understand."

I look at the clock and check the time: 12:45. It takes two hours to drive home from Halifax and I know Mom's waiting by the phone. "I think we should go ahead according to plan."

Dick resumes his post.

I resume mine.

The recording light on the console glows red.

Mom picks up after the first ring. "Hello?"

"Hey, Mom."

"How's it going?"

"It goes."

We both pause for a deep breath.

"Are you ready?" I ask.

"I'm ready," she says.

I try to find a way to take the sting out of what I'm about say. "Well, I always said that I wanted to be just like you—"

"Yes?"

"And I am."

"Oh, honey."

"It's okay. At least now I know."

"Well, you've got a big job ahead."

"Yeah, a lot of work cut out for me."

As we both start to cry, I hear her whisper, "I'm sorry."

I can't bear the thought of her feeling that she's responsible for this. "Don't cry," I insist. "Please don't cry."

On the way to my car, I walk through the Public Gardens, hoping to calm my nerves before the long drive home. When I pause to sit on a bench on the walking path near Griffin's Pond, my thoughts turn to Brian.

It's only been five weeks since his death, and I'm struggling not to feel as if today's news isn't just a painful continuation of a long nightmare.

I'd already made the decision that I wasn't going to insert his death into the documentary, for a thousand different reasons—it was still too raw, too complicated, too much to process. Also, it simply wasn't part of the story I wanted to tell. *How am I going to explain all this to the Kid?*

Watching the midday sun dance on the surface of the water, I think of the example my mother has set. Through her cancer, and through every struggle she's ever faced, she's always chosen to look ahead and make the most of every day. It's what our ancestors had done for generations in the face of this disease. Now that I've been given the rare opportunity of knowing my fate, it's up to me to make the best of it. As Mom would say, *It's just another opportunity.*

Date: Wednesday, May 15, 2002

Subject: understanding the blue gene

Dear Pumpernickel Schnicklefritz,

Grandpa and I thought you might be a little worried about the results of your mom's tests. So far we know that your mom, two of her cousins, and I have this gene that I call "blue."

The gene tells doctors that we are very strong resilient people who could have certain things happen to them. So a group of special doctors got together and decided on some super-duper tests for us to have once a year to keep us well year after year. Isn't that wonderful? We all are now very healthy and we want to stay this way, so we do just what the doctors tell us is important for us to do.

Do you remember a time ago when we were together and we said no matter what, we would always love each other and always tell the truth? Well trust me when I say that your mom is number-one-super-colossal healthy, OK?

Grandpa and I would like to know more about your art class and all about baseball when you start practice.

More rain on my garden tomorrow. The seeds keep washing away. Can you think of a solution for that?

Happy face in the morning.

Love, Lala and Pa.

Xoxoxoxo

Once one understands a disease, it's only a matter of time
before that disease is conquered. I have a lot more than
hope. I'm absolutely confident that there will be progress.
　　　—Dr. Bert Vogelstein, Dan David Prize lecture, 2018

44.

By Reputation

Scots Bay, Nova Scotia, June 18, 2018

3:55 P.M.

It's five minutes before my phone interview with Dr. Bert Vogelstein,
head of the Ludwig Cancer Center at Johns Hopkins University.
Once I've got him on the line, I'll have just thirty minutes to ask him
everything I want to know about his research, specifically as it per-
tains to Lynch syndrome and Family G.

He'd agreed to the conversation months ago, and I've been cram-
ming for it. After wading through a binder full of research papers,
interviews, and articles, and watching every video of his lectures
I could find, I finally feel as if I'm starting to understand his contributions to the field of modern cancer genetics.

I've come up with a set of questions I can ask in any order, precise
enough to get the information I seek, yet still open enough to allow
for unexpected tangents. My approach is closely based on lessons I
learned from a seasoned jazz piano player I'd sung with in university,
a master of improvisation. "If you know a song's structure, you can
anticipate the changes. Once you can dance with those changes, you've
got room for serendipity."

Taking a deep breath, I pick up the phone.

AM: Just a quick question before we start, would it be all right if
I recorded our conversation?

BV: Yeah, no problem.

AM: Excellent, thanks. Should I get right to it?

BV: Sure, get right to it.

AM: In my email, I explained that I'm currently working on what
I call a "genetic memoir." It traces not only my personal experiences with Lynch syndrome, but also my family's very long history
with it. I'm actually a descendant of what's referred to in medical
literature as Family G.

BV: Yes. Of course. Warthin's Family G.

AM: Yes. That's right, and the seamstress who told him about her
family was my great-great-aunt.

BV: Oh, is that right?

His calling us "Warthin's Family G" makes me flinch. I know
he's speaking scientifically, from a historical point of view, but
I doubt I'll ever get another chance to share Pauline's side of things
with him. Before I ask my first question, I change course to set the
record straight.

AM: She was my great-grandmother's older sister, so I've been
tracing that part of the family's history and writing about her contributions to Warthin's work. She's often mentioned as a footnote
in medical literature, but she was actually the one who compiled
the family's pedigree. She introduced Warthin to her relatives and

helped him collect family histories for about twenty-five years before she passed. Since her part in the research has been over-looked, I've decided to tell her story as well as my own.

BV: That's great. I often presented a picture of her early on in my career, when I started out, talking about doing research, talking about "the seamstress." I know her well by reputation, I guess.

My heart skips a beat.

AM: Oh, good. Does that mean you have a picture of her?

I can't imagine how he would've gotten one, but I have to ask.

BV: No. I just used an old image of a seamstress to represent her. I find that pictures help get the point across. They're more memo-rable than words.

AM: And when you were talking about her, what was the point you were trying to illustrate?

BV: The point I was trying to make was that the hereditary nature of cancer has been known for over a century but only recently was it possible to identify the cause. Family G was one of the first, if not the first, example of an unquestionable relationship of cancer to genetics.

From here I ask a couple of questions about his early research. Even though it's been twenty-five years since he first teamed up with Henry, his memories are both precise and fond—from Henry's freezer full of DNA to Hai Yan's innovative technique for ferreting out the mutation. It's clear he feels a sense of residual wonder at his team's accomplishments.

BV: We worked ridiculously hard to try to identify the gene. Now, it seems so primitive, what we did then, because you can do this in a day now, once you know the location the gene is in, or if not a day, in a few weeks. Back then it was really quite difficult. Even now, those kinds of mutations can be very difficult to discover, even with next generation sequencers. This technique is not something that can be routinely done, but when you have a really important case, like this was, and you're willing to devote the energy and time to do it, it can be illuminating.

I'm struck by the level of dedication that he and his team maintained throughout the process, and everything that's led to their place on the long, serendipitous continuum that leads from Pauline to me. *What if they'd given up?*

AM: I have to say, on behalf of my entire family, thank you. Your work has saved lives. Because of you, people in my family have had genetic testing done and then gone on to have screenings that led to early detection. My eldest brother had a colonoscopy when he was fifty that revealed a small tumour, and because we knew the family history and because of your test, a surgeon immediately performed a subtotal colectomy and my brother has had a great life since then. He's even competed in triathlons.

BV: That's great to hear! I appreciate your telling me. You know I hardly ever get any reports like that back. I just do the work.

AM: Oh, well you should also know that I'm a previvor, an unaffected carrier. I was one of the earliest members of Family G to get tested, and I've had screenings every year with no sign of colorectal cancer, so far. I had a hysterectomy a while back as a preventative measure and I'm very happy and healthy. For my family, the genetic test was truly a miracle, because we'd suffered a century's worth of living and dying and immeasurable sadness, but we never gave up hope. I've got nothing but praise for you and your lab and all the work that you do.

BV: Nobody ever says anything, so it's nice to hear that we actually helped.

To date, over one hundred cancer cell genomes have been sequenced, most of them at Johns Hopkins. Through his decades of research, Vogelstein has crafted a medical legacy that has led from the development of genetic testing for hereditary cancers to immune checkpoint therapies (treatments that help the body recognize and attack cancer cells). He, and other genetic researchers like him, foresee a future in which personalized medicine will be tailored to an individual's unique genome. In the meantime, Vogelstein's got his sights fixed on the early detection of eight common cancers through a simple blood test called CancerSEEK. The test simultaneously evaluates levels of eight cancer proteins and the presence of cancer gene mutations from circulating DNA in the blood. Vogelstein believes that the present war on cancer is far too focused on retaliation. "Early detection is undervalued, underfunded and under-researched in cancer investigations. If we can get society to appreciate the value and historical precedent for this kind of research, we can change what we're doing now for the better and actually be victorious against these diseases."

As we spend the next few minutes talking through the future of genetics in medicine, I ask him where he feels Lynch syndrome fits in the history of medicine.

BV: Certainly the Lynch syndrome story has incredible lessons for cancer in general. Sadly, there are still some even after all these years who doubt that cancer is a genetic disease. The Lynch story, I think, in a very scientific way, closes the book on those doubts. If you have a patient with lots of mutations in their DNA, they are much more likely to develop cancer. It's very similar to smoking, right? The more you smoke, the more you're likely to get cancer. Here, the more mutations you have, the more likely you are to get cancer, and the only thing that the Lynch syndrome gene does is increase mutation rate. It does nothing else.

Making that connection proved cancer is a genetic disease, beyond a shadow of a doubt.

Glancing at my phone, I see our time is nearly up.

AM: Before we go, I'd like to know how you maintain the kind of atmosphere in the lab that fosters creativity and a collaborative approach.

BV: It's not really an issue if you have the right people. All of us realize we have this incredible opportunity both with the technologies that are available and with the generous funding that we receive. Everyone in our lab is there because they want to do something important for other people. They just can't wait to start their day and help, and possibly make a contribution.

But there are hard days too, there are periods, years that all scientists go through in which they are embarking on a discovery. That's not so much fun. But if you have this vision that yes, there really is a gene and you're gonna find it come hell or high water, you eventually do. And that's the way it was with Family G. It took from 1993 to 2000 to find that mutation—seven years. I told you the strategy that worked, but I didn't tell you about all the strategies that failed to reveal the mutation. [He laughs.] They never get published. The post docs and students and everybody else that works so hard at it—there's no award for failure in science. It's very unusual that you get a true Eureka moment, when you have an idea and it actually turns out to be right. But there's also no dearth of motivation, as you can see. It took seven years, but we would've worked on it for another seven, or more, until we found it.

AM: I'm so glad you did. I can't thank you enough.

45.

Go for Launch

Wolfville, Nova Scotia, February 14, 2006

I'm standing backstage in an old community theatre, about to read from my first novel. The house lights haven't dimmed yet, so I can see the place filling up—a mix of friends, family, townsfolk and university students—dozens of kind-hearted human beings there to witness my crazy dream come true. Ian and the boys (now twelve and four) are sitting in the front row surrounded by our closest friends—a merry band of painters, writers, actors, and their kids—kindred spirits who've all chosen to pursue a life in the arts.

Everyone who's supported me on this journey is here, except for my mom.

After the local bookseller makes an introduction, I walk on stage and stand behind a podium. Once the audience is quiet, I deliver a short speech.

"I want to thank you all from the bottom of my heart for being here tonight. And since you're such a lovely crowd, I'd like to ask you for a little favour before I begin my reading.

"My mother, who attended countless piano recitals, high school musicals, university concerts and coffeehouse gigs throughout my life, can't be here tonight. She's currently recovering from surgery for colon cancer and is about to start a series of chemo treatments that will take nine months to complete.

"Since she's not with us, I'm hoping that if I call her on my cell phone you'll be kind enough to help me let her know I'm thinking of her?"

Peering out across the dark theatre I can see people enthusiastically nodding.

"All right then," I say. "Here's how it's going to go. You stay quiet until I've got her on the line, then when I give you the signal we'll all shout, "Hi, Mom!"

We try a practice run to make sure we're all on the same page, then I ask for silence.

The phone rings twice before Mom picks up.

"Hello?"

"Hey, Mom."

"Hey, schnicklefritz!" She sounds surprised. "Isn't tonight your big night?"

"It is," I reply. "But it didn't feel right without your being a part of it, so I thought I'd round up a few friends to call and say hi."

Holding out my phone, I cue the crowd to do their thing and a collective shout of a full house rings through the theatre. "HI, MOM!"

When I put the phone back to my ear I can hear her giggling.

"I love you, Mom."

"I love you too, kiddo."

"I'd talk longer, but I've got this thing I've got to do. I'll call you when I'm done, okay?"

"You'd better."

I'd gone home for her surgery a few weeks before the book launch, and I'd been worried about her ever since. They'd discovered a tumour at her annual colonoscopy and further tests had revealed that the cancer had already spread to her lymph glands. She'd had a couple of other strikes against her as well—one was that she was fourteen years older than the last time she'd had cancer (the Big C at seventy-two is far different than at fifty-eight); and the other was that the surgeon had insisted on removing all but a few centimetres of her colon. "It's the gold standard for Lynch syndrome patients these days," she'd declared with resolute confidence.

Gold standard or not, it'd put her in a world of hurt.

Her body hadn't adjusted well to her missing colon. She'd found it nearly impossible to eat or sleep and she'd been in a massive amount of pain. It'd taken all my strength to leave her and head back to Canada. But she'd insisted: "You go get that book of yours off the ground. And I'll get this old body to behave. We'll meet back here in the fall for one heck of a party."

Writing the novel had been my way of coping after I'd gotten the test results. While struggling with whether or not I wanted to have another child, I'd immersed myself in a fictional world that revolved around pregnancy, childbirth and motherhood, constructed from the stories the women in my community had told me about the midwife who'd once lived in my house. As the years went by, and each birthday passed (thirty-four, thirty-five, thirty-six, thirty-seven), the answer had come clearer, but it had been my mother who first declared, "That book's your baby." She was right. It'd been something I could nurture into existence while mourning the loss of a future I'd thought was sure. For a while, I'd been convinced that my mother viewed the novel as nothing but a selfish distraction standing between her and another grandchild. But she'd become my biggest fan. I'd sent her a few chapters at a time, and as she read she discovered my story between the lines. "This is what you were meant to do," she'd said. "Never doubt it."

Just after the Wolfville launch, as I embark on my first book tour across Canada, Mom has a port installed in her chest for her chemo. I call her every night while I'm on the road to describe the places I'm seeing for the first time: the majestic Canadian Rockies west of Calgary, the verdant Pacific coast of Vancouver, the steep streets and colourful clapboard buildings of St. John's, Newfoundland. In return, she tells me tales of the people she's met during her treatments: a young mother with a new baby, a woman who used to work in Dad's office, an elderly gentleman who loves crossword puzzles. Two weeks into the tour, she breaks the news to me that my eldest brother, Skip, has also been diagnosed with colon cancer and that he'll soon be going under the knife. He's only fifty.

"Thank God they found it when they did," Mom says. "It was a very small tumour and nothing had spread, so he may not even have to have chemotherapy."

"That's good," I say, reeling.

Several months after I'd gotten my results, my brother Doug had tested positive for the gene, but Skip still hadn't taken the plunge to get tested. He had, however, signed up for a routine colonoscopy when he turned fifty. That's what had saved him.

"They'll run a test to confirm it," Mom adds, "but I think it's safe to say that he's got the marker too. Bearing that, I convinced him he needed to have a consultation with my surgeon since he's one of the few docs in the area who's up to date on the latest recommendations for Lynch syndrome."

"How'd that go?"

"Skip was a bit shocked by the thought of having his colon removed, but when the doc told him that one resection would probably lead to another and another, he smartened up."

"So he's having the same surgery as you?"

"Yes."

I can't imagine it. Skip is an intelligent, hyper-confident, athletic father of two teenagers who never seems to have a care in the world. Picturing him in a hospital bed with tubes sticking out of his body is nearly impossible.

"He's going to be fine," Mom says. "As will I."

"All right," I say, unsure of everything.

46.

When Silence Is Betrayal

Scots Bay, Nova Scotia, June 30, 2018
Protests are being held across the United States today in support of the Families Belong Together movement. It's good to see so many people filling the streets and squares, but it's also heartbreaking to think of why they are there—the "zero tolerance" immigration policy Trump put in place last month. Children of parents who are seeking refugee status are being taken away and held in detention camps with no clear plan for them to be reunited with their families. Mothers are being told by immigration officials at the US-Mexico border that their children need to be escorted away for a hot meal and a bath, and the children are never brought back. Footage of the camps shows kids sleeping on gym mats on concrete floors and confused, crying toddlers locked up in enclosures that look an awful lot like dog run cages at the pound.

On average, forty-five migrant children are being taken from their families each day. There are at least one hundred "shelters" for these children across the US in seventeen different states. Currently there are nearly twelve thousand kids being detained. A few of the shelters have been designated as "tender age" camps for toddlers and infants. A federal judge has recently ordered the Trump administration to take steps to reunite these children with their families (children under five, in the space of two weeks; children five and older, within thirty days). To date, only a handful of kids have been returned to their parents.

Many are comparing these actions to the way parents and children were separated during WWII in Germany and calling Trump a

Nazi. I wonder how many US citizens know of the country's shameful history when it comes to eugenics and how it inspired the horrors carried out by Hitler? There are so many frightening parallels between this moment in US history and Pauline's time. Trump constantly uses the language of the eugenicists, insisting that immigrants (who he often refers to as "criminals" or "animals") will "invade our borders" and "infect our country." His first attorney general, Jeff Sessions, publicly stated a desire to return to the Johnson-Reed Immigration Act of 1924, an act that prompted President Coolidge to declare as he signed it: "America must stay American." Sessions' justification for his attachment to that old bill sounds like the propaganda of the 1920s: "The percentage of foreign-born in America is about as high as it's ever been and it's surging more."

What he doesn't mention is that the act was engineered to restrict immigration of multiple ethnic and racial minorities with an eye towards the blatant support of the American eugenics movement's agenda. The House Committee on Immigration and Naturalization at the time even appointed an "Expert Eugenics Agent" who gave "scientific" testimony stating that certain ethnic groups were "socially inadequate" and likely to become a "public burden" that would pollute the American gene pool with intellectually and morally defective citizens.

A recently leaked draft of an executive order uses similar language: "immigration laws must ensure the United States does not welcome individuals who are likely to become a burden to taxpayers."

Such white identity politics aren't exclusive to the Oval Office. Yesterday I watched a video of white nationalists chugging milk from plastic jugs to advance the anti-immigrant message: "If you can't drink milk, you have to go back." In it, a dozen or so shirtless white males take turns flexing and grunting in front of the camera, milk running down their chins as they spew hateful ideology based on the racist misuse of genetics. At one point, a participant approaches the camera and boldly sneers, "An ice cold glass of pure racism." The milk emoji has recently gained popularity among white nationalists on Twitter. Trump supporters are now bringing jugs and cartons of milk to his rallies. They all foolishly believe that their ability to digest lactose proves their superiority.

It's just one of several pseudo-scientific narratives neo-Nazi and white nationalist groups have been spreading on alt-right news sites and web forums on the internet. By cherry-picking short passages and illustrations from scientific papers, they filter geneticists' findings through the lens of racism in support of their cause. Forgetting the past truly has doomed us to repeat it.

How many people believe in this hateful rhetoric?

Is there anything scientists can do to fight against the blatant misappropriation of their work?

As of this morning, 23andMe executives have volunteered to take DNA samples from the parents and children who have been separated by Trump's zero tolerance policy. At first blush it seems like the testing could be a wonderful win for the families and for science. It would certainly make reuniting them easier. But what happens to that information and those DNA samples afterward? Does ICE take possession of the resulting database? Or the US government? Or 23andMe?

I truly believe that researchers like Dr. Lynch and Dr. Vogelstein are driven by their desire to help people like my family live long, productive lives. I also want to believe that the geneticists at 23andMe are acting with good intentions. But even if that's the case, it still seems that there will always be others (politicians, special interest groups, institutions and corporate executives included) who will do whatever it takes to bend science to their will. If goodness is to prevail, we must never abandon our defence of truth.

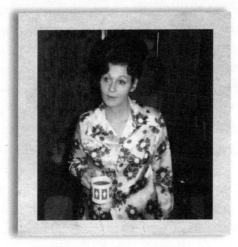

"We'll have a real party."
—Mom

47.

Lost

Broadripple, Indiana, October 2006
The fall after my first novel is published, I take my family home to visit my parents. Together we throw a literary bash at a beautiful little bookstore in Broadripple, Indiana, where siblings, cousins, and friends from high school and university crowd into the shop for an evening of celebration. My cousin Lacie wobbles in the door, pregnant with her first child.

Seeing the smile on my mother's face as I read from my work is like feeling the sun kiss my cheek on the first warm day of spring.

She'd gone all out for the occasion—baking treats, getting her hair done. She'd seemed in her element, but by the end of the evening, I can tell the party has taken a toll.

She's different than the first time she'd had cancer. Her once bouncy dark hair is now thin and wiry and completely grey. Her muscles are atrophied, her skin paper thin; she's more skeletal than sinewy under her clothes. Her hands are always cold, so she wears gloves to get things out of the freezer. She tells me, "Sometimes I leave them on for hours. I can't remember the last time I felt warm." She gets dizzy spells and runs out of breath walking from one end of the house to the other. She can't eat half the things she cooks for Dad without paying for it later. She gets up several times a night to go to the bathroom. She hasn't had a full night's sleep in months and has started taking opium tincture to control her bowel movements and her pain.

"Laudanum?" I ask. The transformation of my mother into an ill-fated character from a Victorian penny dreadful is complete.

"I hate taking the stuff, but it's the only thing that works. I think I'd be dead without it."

In a quiet moment alone with me, she admits she's depressed. "I just don't understand why I haven't licked this yet. Skip's doing so well."

My brother is twenty years younger than she is, and he hadn't had to suffer through nine months of chemo. "What does your doctor say about it?" I ask.

"She says I should be patient, give it time."

There's a hesitancy in her voice that I've never heard before. It leaves me wondering if she's told the doctor (or anyone) how bad she truly feels.

January 21, 2007

My regular Sunday evening chat with Mom is later than usual since the Indianapolis Colts are vying for the AFC Championship against the New England Patriots, and both Dad and Mom are glued to the game to the very end.

It's nearly midnight when she finally checks in. I can hear my dad and brother whooping it up in the background.

"I take it the Colts won?" I ask.

"How'd you guess?"

It sounds as if she's out of breath.

"You feeling all right, Mom?"

"I'm just really beat. I haven't felt up to snuff for a couple of days."

"Maybe you should have Dad take you in to emerg?"

"Nah," she replies. "The last thing I want is to get stuck in the ER in the middle of the night. I've got a doctor's appointment first thing tomorrow to check my potassium. I'm sure she'll give me something to fix me up."

"What's wrong with your potassium?"

"It's been out of whack for a little while now." She's working hard to sound nonchalant.

"Is it dangerous?" I ask.

"It'll be fine, kiddo. I think I'm gonna turn in now and get some rest. Can I call you tomorrow?"

"Sure, Mom," I say. "Sweet dreams. Happy face in the morning. I love you."

January 22, 2007

When the phone rings, I'm still in my pajamas.

"I wonder who that is," Ian asks, poking at the fire in the wood stove. "No one ever calls this early."

I skitter across the cold linoleum floor and pick up the receiver. "Hello?"

"Ami?"

"Dad?"

"Are you sitting down?" he asks. I can tell he's been crying. "Can you sit down, honey? I need you to sit down."

"Okay, Dad," I say. "I'm sitting. What's wrong?"

"Your mom's gone. She died in her sleep."

The shock hits me so hard I can't speak.

"Are you there, Ami?" he asks. "Can you hear me?"

"Yeah, Dad." *Why didn't I insist on talking to him last night? I should've convinced him to take her to the hospital.*

Voice shaky with grief, he says, "She'd been sleeping in the extra room because she didn't want to bother me when she got up at night. This morning when I woke up she was still in bed. I called to her and she didn't answer. When I went to her, she was cold, she wasn't breathing. Her mouth was open, like she was scared, surprised." He starts to sob. "What am I going to do without her?"

I can't bear the thought of him being alone.

"Is there anyone there with you?"

"Skip's on his way. And the coroner should be here soon."

"I'm going to stay on the line until someone comes, okay?"

"Okay."

"And then I'll get on a plane and come home."

January 24, 2007

After two cancelled flights and a series of hellish delays in Boston, I finally walk through the door of my childhood home with my eldest son. A nasty winter storm had raced up the eastern seaboard and swept through the Maritimes, making travel nearly impossible. I'm thankful Ian has decided to stay in Nova Scotia with our youngest. Changing flights and chasing after lost luggage for two was hard enough.

My siblings are all there when I arrive, sitting with Dad and sorting through old photos to display at the funeral home during the visitation and memorial service. When I see Dad, I instantly start to cry.

My mother had always been the first person I'd seen whenever I'd walked into the house, and the first to embrace me. *I can't believe she's gone.*

"Come pick out your favourites," my sister says, holding out a ragged shoebox stuffed with pictures.

"I don't know if I can," I say, reaching for a tissue from the box that always sat by Mom's chair. Her recliner is empty, but her pet schnauzer is curled up asleep in a dog bed on the floor beside it.

My heart breaks as my son sits on the floor next to the pup and strokes its soft fur.

"She misses your grandma something terrible," my dad tells him. "And so do I."

I sit and hold Dad's hand until he falls into a restless nap in his chair. Then I get up to walk around the house.

Doug moves to follow me, but my sister says, "Let her go."

Everything in the bathroom still smells like Mom. The scent of cocoa butter lotion mixed with her favourite perfume clings to the terrycloth hand towels and lingers in the air. Objects are where she left them—a grocery list on a pad of paper by the phone, a half-read novel splayed face down on the coffee table, a spool of blue thread with a needle tucked cockeyed through its centre.

The door to the room where she died is closed. I don't open it. Instead, I force myself to confront the most difficult room of all—the heart of the home she made for us—her kitchen.

When I get there, I find my son standing next to the sink, his face streaked with tears.

"Oh, kiddo," I say, folding him in my arms. "She loved you so."

As I hold him, I look at all the things that have been there since my youth—the copper jelly moulds and old china plates that ring the room above the cupboards, the caddy of wooden spoons and rubber spatulas on the counter by the stove, the pair of shot glasses by the sink—one for Mom, one for Dad. In recent years she'd begun using them to sort their daily meds. Hers has a flock of Canada geese in flight etched in it, circling the rim.

Spying a small bottle of opium tincture sitting next to it, I break from my son to pour its contents down the drain.

"Are you hungry?" I ask, sounding like my mother.

"Kinda," my son says. "I don't know."

"How about we split a PB&J?" *That's my girl,* Mom whispers in my ear.

"Sure," my son replies.

I locate the peanut butter and grape jelly, then I grab Mom's bread basket from the top of the fridge. Pulling a loaf of sourdough out of it, I discover an old cookie tin. I instantly know what's in it. Each Christmas, she always hid a few lebkuchen away to have with her morning coffee after the holidays were over. Lifting the lid on the tin, I remove a cookie and take a bite. It's stale and crumbles down the front of my blouse, but finding it here, today, feels like a gift. My world will never be the same without her, yet somehow my mother is still able to nourish and comfort me.

Cancer is still a word that strikes fear into people's
hearts, producing a deep sense of powerlessness.

—Angelina Jolie

48.

The Angelina Effect

Scots Bay, Nova Scotia, May 14, 2013
This morning Angelina Jolie published an op-ed in the *New York
Times* called "My Medical Choice." In it, she writes of her decision as
a BRCA1 carrier to have a double mastectomy to prevent breast
cancer, which killed her mother. By noon, every branch of the media—
television, print, radio, the internet—is buzzing with the news.

Some are using the words "brave" and "courageous" to describe
her decision. Others are saying she's engaging in medical fearmonger-
ing. Her genetic mutation isn't the same as mine, but I deeply empa-
thize with her situation. She says she hopes her story will open the
door to other conversations on genetic testing for hereditary cancers.
I do too. Such discussions are never easy, and neither are the choices
that come with having a positive result.

I'm forty-four and still haven't had a hysterectomy.

My dead mother nags me, *Why the hell not?*

Because I'm scared.

I don't want to have major surgery. I don't want to give up my
womb even though I know it's the smart thing to do. I don't want
Lynch syndrome to dictate what I should do with my body. I've
known the odds are against me for the past eleven years.

Don't let your fear make you stupid, dear.

At first I'd told myself that I wasn't ready to close the door on the possibility of having another child. Then that I was too busy with the boys to be laid up for six weeks post-surgery. After that I'd gone on my first book tour. Then my mother had died. Then I'd written a play followed by another novel. Then my dad had gotten ill and died. Then another book tour had come along, and another novel was in the offing.

There just never seemed to be a right time to surrender my uterus.

Yet it seemed my body was getting tired of waiting for me to make up my mind. Over the past year, my periods had been getting progressively more painful and worrisome. I was spotting between my cycles, and last month, the bleeding had been so heavy that I'd been afraid to leave the house for fear I might pass out. My new gynecologist had warned me at my last appointment that the screening methods for detecting endometrial and ovarian cancers are less than ideal. "Just let me know when you're ready for surgery," he'd said. "We'll get you in right away."

What are you waiting for?

I sit down at my desk and Google the symptoms for endometrial cancer.

Vaginal bleeding not associated with menstrual period.

Pelvic pain.

Pain with urination.

Abnormal cycles: extremely long, heavy or frequent episodes of bleeding.

Fuck.

I can't grab the phone fast enough to call my gynecologist.

A week later, I'm sitting in the waiting room of his office, torn between my fear of cancer and my fear of surgery.

I've paid attention to my body my entire life—I don't smoke. I rarely drink. I eat whole, organic foods whenever possible. I like my uterus, which has shed its lining like clockwork since I was eleven, and carried and nurtured my two sons.

How can I just abandon it?

On the heels of the Angelina Jolie article, a friend who's aware of my status had sent me a link to a video showing a woman who claimed she'd been able to "change her DNA" through meditation. Although my friend meant well, the video had only served to make me feel like a failure.

Snap out of it.

During the appointment, my gynecologist lists the possible complications and risks of a hysterectomy:

Blood clots.

Infection.

Excessive bleeding.

Damage to the urinary tract, bladder, bowel, rectum.

Early onset of menopause, which may lead to: hot flashes, night sweats, disturbed sleep, mood swings, osteoporosis.

If the ovaries aren't removed, ovary failure.

He says, "If you decide to keep your ovaries, I recommend you have your fallopian tubes removed along with your uterus and cervix. Recent studies have shown that certain types of ovarian cancers actually begin in the tubes."

I know that women all over the world have hysterectomies every day, but that doesn't make me any less nervous. All I can remember from my mother's operation is sitting next to her lawn chair in the backyard, grass prickling my bare legs as I held her hand, post-surgery.

Better make up your mind, kiddo, before it's too late.

"When would you like to schedule the operation?" the gynecologist asks, thumbing through his calendar on his desk.

"Is there a rush?"

"No," he says, "but were you going to suggest we wait?"

"Maybe just until I've finished the current draft of my novel."

"When will it be finished?"

"Six months? Maybe longer?"

He shakes his head. "You're forty-four years old. You have Lynch syndrome. Your cycles are becoming more and more abnormal every month. Think of how you'll feel if cancer arrives while you're waiting."

Two days before my forty-fifth birthday, Ian drives me to the hospital for my surgery. I spend most of the trip reminding him of things he already knows. "There's a pot roast in the freezer. If you stick it in the crockpot by 10 a.m., it'll be done by six."

"Your sister says she's already got dinner planned."

Lori had arrived from Michigan the previous night.

"Well, it's there, just in case . . ."

"You're going to be fine," he says. "You know that, right?"

"Yeah," I say, watching the green of the valley roll past my window.

We'd spent the previous afternoon with the boys, harvesting the first honey from our hives. Catching the liquid gold on his finger as it'd poured out of the extractor, Ian had offered me the first taste. Nothing had ever been sweeter.

Leaning close, I kiss his cheek. "Thank you," I whisper in his ear.

"What for?"

"For our life."

Now get in there and let the nice doctor give you a hysterectomy.

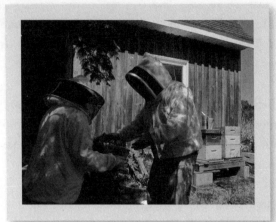

49.

Soulmates

Scots Bay, Nova Scotia, July 2, 2018
It's just shy of 6:00 a.m. when Ian rolls out of bed and says, "I'm going to get the bees."

I kiss him goodbye. "I'll be waiting."

In the space of the next hour, he'll drive to an apiary in the Annapolis Valley and fetch a pair of "nucs" (small wooden boxes, each fitted with four frames of comb, a home for approximately fifteen thousand honey bees, and a queen). Avoiding sharp turns and sudden stops, he'll carefully bring them home so we can acclimate them to their new hives. It will be an all-day affair, requiring patience and care every step of the way.

This is our fifth year of keeping bees, but the first time since we began that we're starting over from scratch.

Even before we'd gotten word from the beekeeper that the nucs would be ready today, we'd been preparing for the bees' arrival. Cleaning two old hives from top to bottom, we'd scraped away old bits of comb and propolis, then scorched the insides with a blowtorch to rid the

wood of any fungus, mites or disease. Together, we'd walked the property to find what we'd hoped would be a better location for the hives,
finally settling on a spot between the south-facing side of the barn and
a small pond that's home to water lilies, duck weed, robber frogs and
salamanders. When they were little, our sons used to sit there for hours,
dragonflies zooming over their heads as they'd watched tadpoles dart
and wiggle their way to gangly-legged maturity.

When Ian gets back, I run out to greet him. I watch as he gently
places the nucs in front of their respective hives.

Despite my husband's thoughtful care, the bees are vigorously
buzzing inside their small quarters, disoriented from their recent journey. "We should let them settle," Ian says. "So they can calm down
before we re-home them."

I nod as we move away and let them rest.

The morning is clear and warm, with no sign of fog on the Bay.
It's my parents' anniversary. Wandering through the yard, I pick a
small bouquet in Mom and Dad's honour, peonies, roses, day lilies and
the last blossoms from a late-blooming lilac called "Miss Kim." Taking
them to my studio, I set them in a vase on my desk.

Reaching for a wooden box that's sitting next to the flowers, I lift its
lid and pick out a bundle of yellowed envelopes—the letters my parents
had written to each other while my dad was in the navy. Although I'd
read a few of them on different occasions, I've never read all of them in
one sitting. Loosening the pale blue ribbon tied around them, I organize
the letters by postmark: December 1951 to late June 1954.

After Mom's passing, Dad had encouraged my sister and me to go
through her things and take whatever we wanted. Both of us felt as if
Mom might walk through the bedroom door at any moment and
scold us for raiding her closet, but we'd done our best.

I'd wound up with an odd mix of things that wouldn't mean much
to anyone else—a black double-breasted blazer she'd sewn herself, a

pair of silver dancing shoes, a few trinkets from her jewellery box, and her pair of black patent pumps, which I'd worn to her funeral because the airline lost the bag that'd held my shoes.

While sorting through the things in her dresser, I'd found the Family G registry from Dr. Lynch, which I'd kept, and the love letters, which I'd promptly given to Dad.

Clutching them in his hand he'd said, "I should probably just burn them."

"Oh, Dad, no. You don't really mean that, do you?"

"Your mom's gone and I already know what they say. When I go, there won't be anyone left who cares about them."

"I'll care," I'd said. "They're part of my history too."

Stowing them in the drawer of the coffee table with the remote controls and a stack of ancient TV guides, he'd said, "I'll think about it." I was certain I'd never see them again.

Four years later Dad was diagnosed with terminal lung cancer. Within a month of his diagnosis, I was sitting at his bedside in my hometown hospital. During the last week of his life, my siblings and I stayed with him in shifts around the clock, sometimes in pairs, sometimes alone. Whenever I had solo duty, I'd read him his favourite poetry (the Roberts: Frost and Service) and sing him songs he'd taught me in my youth ("In the Garden," "Blue Water Line," "500 Miles"). When he slept, I'd pick at the edits of my second novel as much as my brain would allow. I managed to write Dad into a scene in the form of a fictional German grocer on the Lower East Side of New York in 1871. Our hours together were dwindling, but I was determined to keep him alive in the pages of my book.

Shortly after his passing, I'd returned to Nova Scotia, leaving the bulk of the task of sorting through the house to my eldest brother, Skip. A few months later he sent a large parcel containing a tea set that my dad had brought back from Japan and most of our family photos. Tucked inside a shoebox with a bunch of loose slides was the bundle of letters. A note attached in Dad's handwriting read: "For Ami."

❧

Now, as I wait for the bees to settle, I read the letters from start to finish.

With every page, I discover countless gems and revelations. Most striking among them is that even when so young—Mom was eighteen and Dad was twenty—their thoughts and the cadence of their sentences are instantly recognizable to me. Mom is already Mom, and Dad is clearly Dad.

In her graceful way, Mom didn't take any shit. She writes plainly, but eloquently, about her philosophy of trust. The rules were clear: there was to be no messing around with her heart.

Dad is his forthright, funny self, sometimes poetic enough to be the Shakespeare of the Shiawassee River Valley:

> Have you ever compared the condition of the weather and the
> type of day it is with someone you know? If you have, you under-
> stand what I mean when I say this beautiful autumn day reminds
> me of you. It's so pure and sweet that it's almost intoxicating.

From the start, they write in terms of the future they'll share. They encourage one another to recount the mundane details of their days, just as they'd later do at the family supper table every night of my childhood. Dad writes of the planes he has to test and repair and look after—Beechcrafts, SNJs. Mom writes of stealthily knitting socks for him during biology class, and of her scheme to send his favourite cake to him for his twenty-first birthday.

Letter by letter, line by line, they dream up a life of happiness, one that looks astoundingly similar to the one they worked so hard to make for us kids.

Just as I finish reading, Ian comes in with our two bee jackets in hand and asks, "Ready to suit up?"

I put the letters away. "You bet."

As we carefully transfer the frames from the nucs to the hives, Ian takes a brief moment to inspect each one to get a feel for the bees' overall health and temperament. The better we know them, the easier it will be to care properly for them.

Once the bees are settled, we remove our gear and sit next to each other on the ground near the hives to watch them take their first orientation flights. Ian holds my hand as we observe their soaring paths in the ecstatic blue of the summer sky. Some venture out to sip water from the moss at the edge of the pond, others nuzzle the petals of the wild roses that skirt the side of the barn. How do any of us ever find where we belong? It's a marvel.

If my mother had not said yes to a blind date with my father, I wouldn't have been born.

If I hadn't daydreamed of a boy who could recite Byron, I wouldn't be sitting where I am now, next to Ian. A man who reminds me daily that mindfulness is essential and worry a thief—of time, happiness and heart.

50.

Star Light, Star Bright

Scots Bay, Nova Scotia, July 2018
My fiftieth birthday begins with me chasing after a dream that's still clinging to me as I wake. I grab paper and pen from the bedside table so I can write it down before it slips away.

I'm on the top floor of the Harold Washington Library in Chicago, under the beautiful glass roof of the Winter Garden. I enter a small café where there are only men sitting at the tables. Most are wearing suits. They all stare at me, but don't say anything. I can't tell if they think I don't belong there, or what. I'm uncomfortable, but I decide to find a quiet corner here anyway.

As I walk through the café, a woman approaches (a librarian?) and says, "I've been waiting for you. Please come with me. The music is this way."

I follow.

She leads me down a corridor to another room where there's a fireplace with a large stone mantel and a woman standing next to it playing the violin. The song she's playing has a haunting, beautiful melody. There are other sounds as well—clarinet, accordion, finger cymbals, but I can't see any other instruments and no one else is with us.

I sit down and listen.

After a while, Ian joins me. He hands me a crumpled brown bag. "I'm sorry I didn't wrap it."

"I don't mind. I'm just glad you're here with me."

When I open the bag I find a glass perfume bottle with a black lid. The label on the bottle reads: "Dr. Whynot's Apothecary: Be a Star."

As I unscrew the lid, I inhale the bright scent of whatever's inside.

"Do you like it?" Ian asks.

That's when I remember the perfume oil I'd worn while I was in grad school. I'd bought it from a woman at a boutique where she'd sold tarot cards, crystals and oils that she'd mixed following what she averred were "ancient rites and the phases of the moon." The one I'd faithfully anointed myself with each day had been called "Happiness," because the shopkeeper had said the scent would help draw it into my life.

"Do you like it?" Ian asks again.

"It's perfect."

The rest of the day is spent in the wake of the dream, moving from one happiness to the next.

Youngest Son calls from camp, where he's in the middle of his second year as a counsellor. "I'll be home on the weekend," he says. "Feel like celebrating your birthday all over again?"

"You bet."

Ian and I have brunch in Wolfville, then browse through piles of books and LPs at the local used bookstore and record shop. My day is made when I find a few records that my parents had in their collection: Ella Fitzgerald singing Gershwin; Tony Bennett with Bill Evans; Helen Reddy's *Long Hard Climb*.

Mid-afternoon we head back home to meet Eldest Son and his sweetheart for a walk on the beach and a swim in the Bay. Our old Labrador, Ponyo, even paddles out to join us in the chilly water. After we walk back to the house, Eldest Son presents me with a sculpture he's made for my garden—a joyful, modernist birdbath that's painted in a fantastic array of colours and patterns. It's the first new work of his I've seen since he'd gotten his results.

"I love it," I say, admiring it from every angle.

To me it embodies all that I want for him: hope, joy, passion, life.

After dinner, I sit outside and wait for the first stars to appear. As they wink into my view against the twilight, I think of the lessons I've learned, the stories I've found, the dreams I've chased this past year. I think of my mother, and her mother, and her mother's mother, and of Pauline—dressmaker, keeper of stories, bearer of truth. They, along with Ian and the boys, have formed a constellation in my heart, always with me, ever pointing me towards home.

Soon, I'll need to turn my attention to cake, candles and the matter of a wish. I'd assumed that I'd simply repeat my heartfelt plea from years past: *Not yet.*

But tonight those words feel beside the point. What I want, more than anything else, isn't to hold back fate but to converse with it.

> *When I heard the learn'd astronomer,*
> *When the proofs, the figures, were ranged in columns before me,*
> *When I was shown the charts and diagrams, to add, divide, and measure*
> *them,*
> *When I sitting heard the astronomer where he lectured with much*
> *applause in the lecture-room,*
> *How soon unaccountable I became tired and sick*
> *Till rising and gliding out I wandered off by myself*
> *In the mystical moist night-air, and from time to time*
> *Look'd up in perfect silence at the stars.*
>
> —Walt Whitman

Scots Bay, Nova Scotia, October 24, 2018
Dear Reader,

Today I had my annual colonoscopy.

It was clear.

In my post-scope haze I took a nap, ate some soup and checked my email. Among the messages in my inbox was a note forwarded to me by a certain well-known DNA testing service to which I'd once sent a tube of my spit in order to uncover my ancestral "roots."

From a Relative:
Hello Ami,

My name is Jane Doe.

I recently submitted my DNA to this service and discovered that we are related. I'm sorry I do not know much about the family because I was adopted back when I was born in Michigan in 1964.

I would like to communicate with you to learn about where I come from.

I hope to hear from you soon.

Jane.

I log into the site to see if I can figure out how our DNA matches up. Although I can't tell straightaway how we're related, I can see that Jane shares 1.7 percent of my DNA. That means we likely share a pair of great-great-grandparents. Since she was born in Michigan, I immediately think, *What if she's a part of Family G?*

Dear Jane,

Thanks for reaching out to me. I'd love to get to know you and share some stories.

Welcome to the family.

Let's talk.

ACKNOWLEDGEMENTS

Writing this book required long stretches of solitude that were humbling and essential. Of all the things I've ever written, it demanded my attention in ways that no other work has. And so I begin this note of gratitude with an apology to those dearest to me—Ian, ES and YS, for all the times I acted more stray-cat than human while writing this book. Thank you for believing in me and for sustaining the garden of my soul with your love, laughter, kindness and light. I love you to the moon and back, always.

My love and thanks also go to my siblings—Skip, Doug and Lori, for putting up with the dinner-table monologues of my childhood, for being amazing role models, and for trusting me not to screw this up.

To my extended Family G—those who I grew up with as well as those I've only recently discovered—thank you for being open with your memories and your hearts. Cousin Holly, you are a rock. Cousins Lacie, Chris and Jenna, thanks for sharing your stories and your archives. Cousin Lisa, thanks for the pre-fiftieth pep talk. Cousin Dave, meet me in Ypsilanti, I owe you dinner at Haab's. Niece Anna, there'll be a bag of Montreal bagels on their way to you shortly.

To friends, far and near, your support and encouragement mean the world to me. A million thanks is nowhere near enough.

To Dawn, Marta, Sarah, Jon and Mark—I'm so grateful I met you way back when, and to still call you my friends after all these years.

To Holly, Alan, Chris and Ken—thanks for listening as I talked myself into telling this tale.

To Bree—thank you for kitchen conversations, keeping my cupboard stocked with teas of comfort and dreams, and for loving my son. I'm so glad you're part of our lives.

To Sara H.R.—thank you for walks in mossy groves, conversations about liminal spaces and for reading my fledgling attempts at charting this journey with words.

To the Summer 2017 cast and crew of *Nothing Less!* at the Ross Creek Centre for the Arts: Ken, Robin, Jennifer, Michelle, Chris, Devin, Riel, Vicky, Andrea, Jeff, Burg, Ryan, Graham, Jamie, Dan, Laura and Stephanie. It was an honour to make theatre and music with you. Thank you for bonfires and porch songs, for birthday cake and D&D with Marty, Michaela, and the world's best DM, Ian. You graciously fed my spirit as I readied myself for a year of wild remembering.

This book would never have been written had I not been encouraged to tell a portion of it in radio documentary form by audio producer extraordinaire Dick Miller. I am truly grateful for Dick's brilliant guidance and perfectly posed questions. I couldn't have asked for a better mentor to help me discover the path to my stories and my voice.

That project opened the door to my first one-on-one conversation with Dr. Henry T. Lynch, and began a dialogue that continues to this day. I am eternally grateful for the kindness and wisdom Dr. Lynch has freely shared with me over the years and I stand in awe of his dedication to helping not only my family, but also many others. Henry, your work has changed countless lives for the better.

My gratitude and admiration also go to Dr. Bert Vogelstein of the Ludwig Center at the Johns Hopkins Kimmel Cancer Center, and Dr. Hai Yan, founder of the Yan Lab at the Preston Robert Tisch Brain Tumor Center at Duke University, who both generously took the time to share their parts in the Family G story with me, and to deftly guide me through the complexities of their work. The years they have devoted to discovering and understanding genetic links to hereditary cancers has transformed the shape of science.

Thanks also to Robin Kunkel, Nancy Fritzemeier and Peter Ouillette of the Department of Pathology at the University of Michigan for your time, care and expertise in locating, restoring and imaging century-old tissue samples from Family G.

In addition to conducting interviews with present-day researchers and gathering the many primary source documents mentioned within the text, I read numerous articles and books that informed this work. Chief among them were the following:

"Colon Cancer Germline Genetics: The Unbelievable Year 1993 and Thereafter," by Albert de la Chapelle, *Cancer Research*, Volume 76, Issue 14 (July 2016).

"Found in the Archives: America's Unsettling Early Eugenics Movement," by Rich Remsberg, npr.org (June 2011).

"Harmony in the Lab," by Eugene Russo, *The Scientist*, 14 [17]:19 (September 2000).

"Heredity as Ideology: Ideas of the Woman's Christian Temperance Union of the United States and Ontario on Heredity and Social Reform, 1880–1910," by Riiko Bedford, *Canadian Bulletin of Medical History*, Volume 32, Issue 1 (Spring 2015).

"Historical Aspects of Lynch Syndrome," by Henry T. Lynch et al., *Hereditary Colorectal Cancer*, 2010.

"History of Hereditary Nonpolyposis Colorectal Cancer or 'Lynch Syndrome,'" by Patrick M. Lynch, *Revista Médica Clínica Las Condes*, Volume 28, Issue 4 (July–August, 2017).

"The History of Lynch Syndrome," by C. Richard Boland and Henry T. Lynch, *Familial Cancer*, Volume 12, Issue 2 (June 2013).

"History and Molecular Genetics of Lynch Syndrome in Family G: A Century Later," by Julie A. Douglas, Stephen B. Gruber et al., *JAMA*, Volume 294, Number 17 (November 2005).

"The Rounded Life of Aldred Warthin," by James Tobin, *Medicine at Michigan*, Volume 11, Number 3 (Fall 2009).

"When Racism Was a Science," by Joshua A. Krisch, *The New York Times* (October 2014).

"Aldred Scott Warthin's Family 'G': The American Plot Against Cancer and Heredity (1895–1940)," by Toine Pieters of Utrecht University, in *History of Human Genetics: Aspects of Its Development and Global Perspectives*, 2017.

Alice Hamilton: A Life in Letters, by Barbara Sicherman, 1984.

War Against the Weak: Eugenics and America's Campaign to Create a Master Race, by Edwin Black, 2012.
The Gene: An Intimate History, by Siddhartha Mukherjee, 2017.

Special collections and archives held in various libraries and historical societies also played a large role in my research. My sincerest thanks to the librarians, researchers, archivists and volunteers who maintain the collections at the following institutions: the Bentley Historical Library at the University of Michigan, the Genealogical Society of Washtenaw County, the Washtenaw County Historical Society, the Saline Area Historical Society, the Clarke Historical Library at Central Michigan University and the records office of Forest Hill Cemetery in Ann Arbor.

I could not do what I do without the expert medical care that I've received since my Lynch syndrome diagnosis. Special thanks go to my Nova Scotia "home team" of doctors past and present: Christopher Yoell, Tracy Newhook, Charles Hamm, Richard Stern, Janet MacNaughton, Michael Shaffelburg and Bruce Musgrave, along with all the wonderfully skilled nurses, radiologists and lab techs who look after my health and well-being.

When it comes to the health and well-being of my career, I'd be lost without my stellar agent, Helen Heller, who, with keen wit, savvy and verve, convinced me that the only way to write this tale was through giving the dead a voice. Thank you, Helen, for everything.

I have been blessed to work with the same fabulously talented dream team from Knopf Canada for over a decade. To my editor, Anne Collins, I give my love and gratitude for her literary prowess, unwavering support and generous spirit. I could not have gone on this journey without you. To designer Kelly Hill I send my undying respect and admiration for her astounding ability to always find the perfect vision for my work. From cover to typeface, you never fail to wow me. To Angelika Glover, Ruta Liormonas, Liz Lee, Sarah Smith-Eivemark and Sarah Jackson, thank you from the bottom of my heart for your dedication to minding the details. You ladies rock.

Writing this book meant saying goodbye, again, to several loved ones I'd lost, but it also afforded me moments of dazzling joy as I met them time and again on the page. As I bring my thoughts to a close, I wish to express my deepest gratitude for those who came before I was born and the sacrifices they made for future generations.

To Johannes and Anna Haab, for having the courage to sail across the sea.

To Kathrina, their youngest daughter, for teaching her children to dream.

To Pauline, for her tenacity.

To Tillie, for her strength.

To Alice, for her passion for story.

To Dad, for showing me that love endures all things.

And to Mom, for the countless seeds of wonder you planted in my heart. Your hopes, dreams and love blossom daily in new and unexpected ways in my life. I am proud to be your daughter.

AMI McKAY is the author of three internationally bestselling novels—*The Birth House*, *The Virgin Cure* and *The Witches of New York*—and the recent yuletide novella, *Half Spent Was the Night*. She began her writing career as a freelance radio journalist, and in 2001 wrote and produced a radio documentary, also called "Daughter of Family G," that traced her decision to undergo genetic testing. It won a Silver Medallion at the Atlantic Journalism Awards, was nominated for a Gabriel Award, and aired on both *The Sunday Edition* on CBC Radio and on National Public Radio in the US. Her non-fiction work has also appeared in *ELLE Canada*, *The Independent*, *Canadian Living* and *Chatelaine*. Born and raised in Indiana, McKay now lives in Nova Scotia.

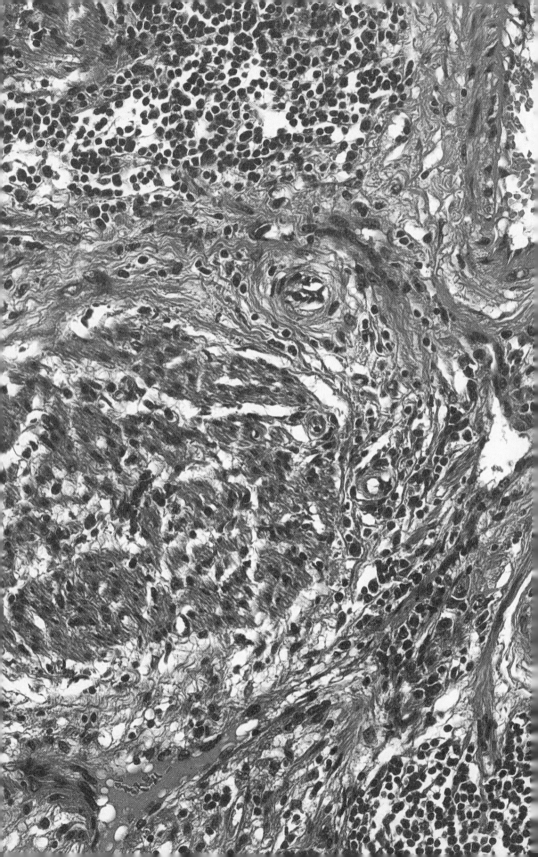